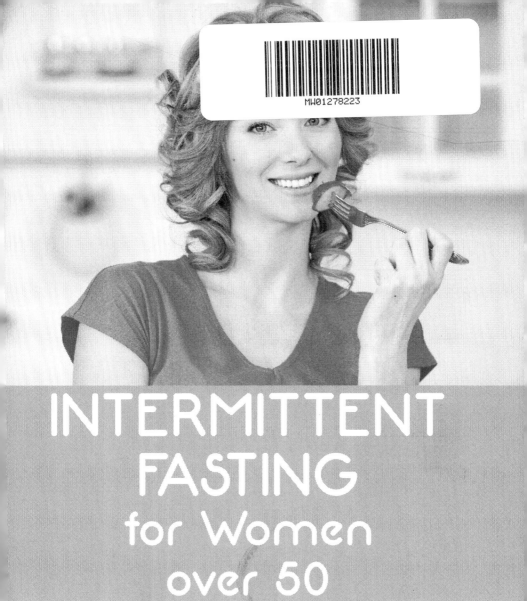

INTERMITTENT FASTING
for Women
over 50

A Guide to Intermittent Fasting and Increasing
Metabolism and Energy Levels. The Best Healthy Way
to Detoxify Your Body and Rejuvenate

Digital Bonus!

Nina Hodgson

Table of Contents

Your Free Gift

Hello and thank you for purchasing the book! I prepared a gift for the readers of:

"Intermittent Fasting for Women Over 50:

A guide to intermittent fasting and increasing metabolism and energy levels. The best healthy way to detoxify the body and rejuvenate. Digital Bonus!"

Click the link and download now the

"Weekly Intermittent Fasting Plan"

https://bit.ly/fastingweeklyplan

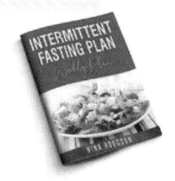

Once you're done reading it, it would be great if you could leave an Amazon review and let other people know about this book as well.

It is very easy to do; you just have to click on this LINK. It will automatically take you to the review section.

Leave a 5-star review:

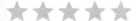

Thanks in advance and enjoy your Intermittent Fasting!

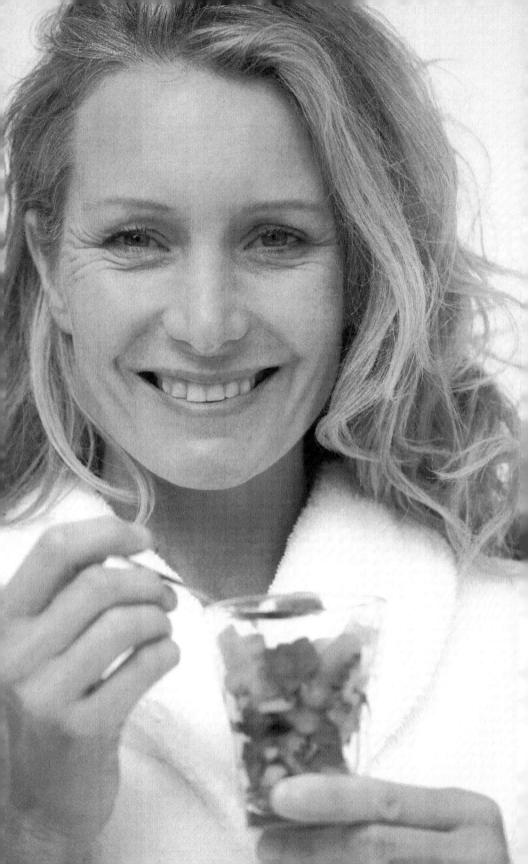

Introduction

Nutritionists have always advised us to eat short and regular meals during the day and never skip them. Now they have changed their minds! They advocate an alternative to diet planning known as intermittent fasting (IF), a meal plan that involves occasional short fasts ranging from 14 to 48 hours and can provide significant health benefits.

Trendy diets abounded in the past and still do today. Diet pills were common in the 1990s. Plus, if you didn't have a juicer when you were in your early 1920s, it meant you didn't care about your well-being. We were advised green tea pods that were supposed to minimize our belly size.

IF is a caloric restriction method that includes feeding intervals and other of fasting. Early research on this eating pattern appears to be quite positive in terms of weight loss, as this diet is similar to other conventional calorie restriction diets.

Each of us has to find a diet plan that suits us best and then just adopt it. Of course, a lot of research is still needed to evaluate the long-term effects and to understand its true role in weight loss, but it is certain that intermittent fasting is a very promising regimen for the treatment of obesity.

Despite this good news, while for some people is healthy, for others it is not. For example, skipping meals for pregnant or breastfeeding women may not be the right way to lose weight. It is also advisable to consult your doctor right from the start of your IF journey if you suffer from gastroesophageal reflux, kidney stones, diabetes, or other medical problems.

This meal plan is a very accessible weight-loss technique because it focuses on meal times rather than avoiding certain ingredients. The IF is easy to follow: you just need to respect the fasting hours without having to worry about the calories you consume.

Nina Hodson fought her weight herself. Although her parents worked in the fields of health and nutrition, she tried to follow many diets, but with poor results: or she could not hold them for long periods, or she regained weight soon after stopping them.

Since she was very young she began to study the subject in-depth, up to obtaining a Masters in Food Education.

With her studies, she understood that each of us must find the right diet, both in relation to what drives us to diet (weight loss, desire to eat healthier), and to our daily rhythms of life.

There seemed to be no suitable diet for her until she tried the IF: it was perfect! She didn't have to count calories, she didn't have to cook special dishes and ingredients and she could also have meals outside, which was common for a busy woman like her.

By reducing obesity, the IF can reduce the risk of heart disease and diabetes, which is not uncommon to find in women of her age. In addition, Nina has decided to collect some healthy recipes to help women to vary their meals and to alternate foods, not neglecting the dietary needs of their fifties: intake of calcium and vitamin D. Since the IF can cause a depletion of minerals and vitamins during the fasting period, you have to drink a lot of water and stay hydrated.

Now, all you have to do is try Intermittent Fasting, following Nina Hodgson's simple but useful tips and experimenting with the recipes she offers you.

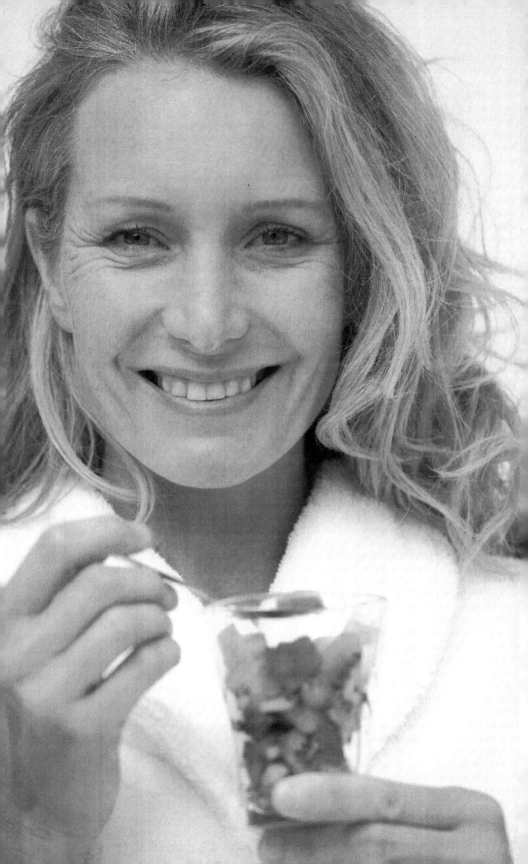

1

Intermittent fasting and how it works

1.1 WHAT IS INTERMITTENT FASTING?

IF is a daily dietary technique that, as the name suggests, alternates fasting and nutrition.

Many studies carried out on the subject indicate that prolonged fasting is a great way to control weight and avoid or even cure certain types of diseases. It should also be added that while most diets focus on limiting food consumption, the IF focuses much more on what to eat.

Fasting for a certain number of hours each day or eating just one meal a few times a week can help the body to metabolize calories and provide great health benefits. Mark Mattson, neuroscientist Ph.D. (Johns Hopkins), has been practicing the IF for 25 years and says that "Our bodies have evolved to be able to hold out for many hours, days or even weeks without eating.

In fact, before humans learned to evolve, they were hunter-gatherers who developed to survive for long periods of time without food. If you think about it, fifty years ago it was easier to maintain a healthier weight. People didn't eat before bed, there were no cell phones, and TV shows ended at 11 pm. Portion sizes were much smaller and most people worked and played outdoors.

Today, TV, telephone, and other sources of content are available 24 hours a day, seven days a week. We stay up late watching videos, playing sports, and talking on the phone. We enjoy all day and we spend half of the night lying down and snacking all the time."

Weight loss is just one of the IF's benefits for a healthy (disease-free) adult. Recent studies in animals and some preliminary studies in humans have shown a decrease in the risk of cancer or a decrease in cancer growth rates due essentially to the following effects of fasting:

- decrease in blood glucose production

- stem cells activated to regenerate the immune system

- balanced nutritional supply

- increased production of tumor-killing cells

1.2 THE SCIENCE BEHIND IF

IF can be done in various ways, but all of them depend on the alternation of regular periods of feeding and fasting. For example, you might consider eating at a specific time of the day and fasting the rest, so eating from 10 am to 8 pm, and fasting from 8 to 10 the next morning. You could also limit yourself to one meal a day for eight hours, twice a week. Don't worry now, later you will find the food plan that best suits your needs, but now let's see what the process that activates the IF is.

According to Mattson, the body reduces its sugar stores and starts burning fat during the fasting hours, this moment is called the metabolic switch. "For many other Americans, who eat during the day, the IF matches the daily diet plan," says Mattson. "If someone eats three meals a day, including snacks and desserts with no physical activity, it is clear that he is getting more than he needs."

With IF, benefits are obtained when the body absorbs all the calories consumed during the previous meal and begins to burn fat. When we feed, more nutritional energy is ingested than is immediately used. This excess energy is set aside by our body for later use, and in this, we are helped by insulin which is the main hormone associated with the storage of food energy.

Insulin increases as we feed, helping to contain extra energy in two different forms: glucose and glycogen. Glucose units (sugar) can be linked together to form glycogen, which is then stored in the muscles or in the liver. However, the storage capacity of carbohydrates is greatly reduced and, if reached, excess glucose is transformed by the liver into fat. De-novo Lipogenesis is the name given to this mechanism (which simply means "making new fat").

Some of this newly produced fat is retained in the liver, but much of it is transported to other parts of the body. Although this is a rather complicated process, there are no limits to the number of fats that can be produced. Therefore, our body operates two important mechanisms of transformation of excess food energy. One is readily available but with minimal "storage" space (glycogen), while the other is more difficult to activate but has almost unlimited storage space (body fat).

This whole process works the other way around when we don't feed. When we are in the fasting period and no energy arrives in the form of food, insulin levels drop, signaling the body to start burning stored energy. Blood glucose decreases because the body must now take it from the depot to burn it and produce energy. Glycogen is the most readily available source of energy and it is broken down into glucose molecules to provide nutrition for other cells in the body. This process will provide enough energy to fuel most of the body's needs for 24–36 hours. After that, the body will have to tap into fat stores (and so break them down) to gain energy.

So we and our body can be in two states: nourishment or fasting. In other words, we are either stockpiling food supplies (increasing supplies and gaining weight) or burning stored energy (decreasing supplies and losing weight), but if nutrition and fasting are balanced, there should be no net weight gain.

If we start feeding the moment we wake up and don't stop until we go to sleep, we spend most of our time in the nourishment state. Therefore, we will begin to gain weight, because we haven't given our body enough time to burn stored dietary fats.

To regain balance or reduce weight, we can increase the average time used to burn food energy.

This is IF.

It encourages the body to use excess fat, and there are no contraindications. It is simply the functioning of our body: either it is in the state of fasting or in the state of nourishment. Simple!

If you eat every three hours, your body will continuously use incoming food resources, never managing to burn your body fat, but rather accumulating it for when you eat less. Remember that if this happens, it means that you are neglecting the balance between the two states (nourishment and fasting) and neglecting the states in which your body can find itself, therefore you neglect the IF.

1.3 INTERMITTENT FASTING CAN HELP LOSING WEIGHT

By following this meal plan, you start consuming fewer calories, which results in a reduction in your overall daily calorie intake. This drastic change in your lifestyle causes major changes in your body that help you lose weight.

During fasting, the body tends to use accumulated body fat as fuel instead of carbohydrate sugars, thereby optimizing insulin synthesis. It has been shown that hormonal changes allow short-term fasting to increase metabolism by 3.6 to 14%. Fasting lowers insulin levels, and the decrease of this enzyme makes stored body fat easily accessible. Then, fat retention is reduced by allowing the body to use the stored fat. For this reason, it is very important and at the same time healthy to keep a low insulin level in order to lose weight.

In the previous paragraph, you read that the food we consume is broken down by enzymes in our stomach which turn into molecules in our bloodstream. Carbohydrates, especially sugars and refined grains (such as white flour and rice), are easily broken down into sugars that our cells use for energy. When the body does not immediately need the excess energy produced, this is stored in our fat cells. Sugar will reach our cells with insulin, a hormone produced in the pancreas that is responsible for transporting glucose from the blood to the organs and cells. Insulin carries fructose into fat cells and holds it there.

Until we eat, our insulin levels drop and our fat cells begin to release the stored sugar to use as energy, thus losing some weight.

This is how IF works!

It encourages insulin levels to drop long enough to burn our weight.

1.4 WHY IS INTERMITTENT FASTING GOOD FOR THE BODY?

Of course, weight reduction is not the only advantage of IF, you would be wrong if you believe this. Below you will read just some of the many benefits your body would have from adopting this type of meal plan. The full list would be truly endless.

1.4.1 IT IS EASIER THAN ANY OTHER DIET

Probably you have done everything possible to follow a diet, ma nothing works. Maybe you've done everything you can to diet, but nothing seems to work. It's not always easy to stick to portion reductions, so losing weight or getting better isn't always a matter of calories. It is more important to change what you eat than how often you eat and this is where the IF focuses the most: it's easy if you understand how to do it.

In addition to this, you need to decide in advance what to eat to stick to the diet, but sometimes you may have a hard time finding the food you like or you may be unconvinced to follow that diet. On the other hand, an intermittent fasting schedule appears to be difficult to follow. For example, a diet typically involves eliminating "bad" ingredients and consuming fewer carbohydrates. Does it seem easy? But what happens when hunger pangs hit you? With IF you can consume even more than you like but at defined intervals. However, try to eat balanced as excess calories can only slow down the weight loss process.

1.4.2 INTERMITTENT FASTING IS LESS STRESSFUL

Imagine starting the day thinking that you have to plan all meals for the day before breakfast. This is the diet routine, which can consume most of the day. Fasting, on the other hand, is easy, transparent, and less tiring. Fasting means consuming one less meal. Therefore, you will not be stressed thinking about what to eat.

1.4.3 IT CAN REDUCE THE RISKS OF ADVERSE HEALTH CONDITIONS

We know that obesity is among the critical causes of health problems. By helping with weight loss and insulin regulation, IF also reduces the possibility of heart attacks and diabetes and all those side effects resulting from excessive calorie consumption and a sedentary lifestyle.

However, it is useful to remember that every physique is different and that IF may not be appropriate for people with health problems.

1.5 HOW TO IMPLEMENT INTERMITTENT FASTING?

After having documented and informed, it's time to understand how to start, and learn correctly what you need to do to practice IF! Now is the time to get started with your routine. Health is the main focus, so make sure you do the following steps before embarking on your journey.

1.5.1 CHOOSE EASY OPTIONS

It is essential, especially if it is the first time. You have to keep doing what makes you feel better. This is the same for meals. It is not a strict diet; you can keep most of your daily meals. Of course, it is good to take the right mix of meals that will help you get the perfect result from your fasting. However, be sure to take in adequate nutrients and fluids and limit the intake of sugar, saturated fat, salt, cholesterol, etc. For starters, no diet sodas, and try to stay well hydrated by drinking plenty of fluids.

Even the reason why you decided to start with the IF is important and makes things so much easier to follow. To begin with, unequivocally identify what your motivations are: to reduce weight, to prevent certain diseases, to live better, or what else?

1.5.2 CONSULT AN EXPERT OR DOCTOR

Like any other diet, if done in the wrong way, it can put your health at risk. So, rather than rush into a fasting regime, find out what's best for your body. This way you can better understand what you can or can't handle. If you have a medical problem, such as diabetes or heart disease, get advice from a professional to get the most benefit without compromising your health.

1.5.3 CALCULATE DAYS AND HOURS

Plan your meal schedule. In this way, you won't run into setbacks and of course, choose your meal times so that they are compatible with your lifestyle.

Days of the week are also important. Most specialists suggest fasting on weekdays, probably because are the days during which we are always full of things to do, so we don't have time to think about hunger and food. Perhaps this is not the case for you, so identify the days that best suit your needs. My advice to start is to adopt limited-time feeding plans rather than follow those where complete fasting is required on certain days of the week.

1.6 INTERMITTENT FASTING PROVIDES ANTI-AGING BENEFITS

During experimenting about the effects of calorie reduction in overweight adults, it was found that calorie reduction increases energy production and reduces the risk of chronic diseases such as heart failure, diabetes, and cancer. In addition, limiting calories was found to also reduce cell damage by helping to preserve stable DNA.

Cell damage and DNA instability are the two main factors to defeat in the fight against aging since weakened and inflamed cells increase the risk of chronic diseases, while aging begins with DNA wear.

Although calories restriction can provide great anti-aging benefits, it is very difficult for most people to follow a diet that includes reducing calorie consumption by 30 to 40 percent and most importantly maintaining it every day for the long term.

This is where IF comes into play: an alternative to calorie restriction because it has been shown to provide the same benefits that prolong life without making unreasonable nutritional demands.

1.7 THE IMPACT OF INTERMITTENT FASTING ON YOUR BODY

Many benefits occur at the molecular level while the body is fasting, even if it is short or sporadic. The following changes, triggered by IF, occur all simultaneously to encourage a healthy and long life:

- Gene expression: changes occur in genes that promote longevity and prevent disease.

- Cells repair: the cells remove more waste that could cause cell damage.

- Protects from oxidative stress: prevents cell damage due to unstable molecules called free radicals.

- Fights inflammation: IF reduces inflammation.

- Hormonal changes: lowering insulin levels prevents diabetes and can increase longevity.

IF allows you to lose weight and abdominal fat, which in turn increases your fitness and eliminates chronic ailments that can prolong your life.

1.8 ANTI-AGING BENEFITS OF CALORIE RESTRICTION

Calorie restriction is the most powerful of all anti-aging treatments. The traditional method involves reducing the intake of calories by 20–40% for long periods of time, which is neither recommended nor not.

According to a very well done article in Clinical Interventions on Aging, titled "Will Eating Less Help You Live Longer and Better?" calories restriction encourages five main, interrelated mechanisms that influence healthy aging:

- Inflammation: NF-kb

- Antioxidants: Nrf2

- Mitochondrial physiology: AMPK / SIRT

- Cell proliferation: IGF-1 and TOR (in particular mTOR)

- Autophagy: foxO

The most significant part of fasting has been found to be the cellular benefits of rest periods. Alicia Galvin, a famous gastrointestinal dietician from Florida, argues that it starts with the mitochondria, the part of the cells that turns food into energy. Their DNA can be depleted when we consume too much of it, but fasting gives them a chance to regenerate, delaying aging on a cellular basis. Regardless of what you consume, fasting will help cells regenerate and heal.

But to reduce weight, Galvin says that the only approach to get the most out of fasting is to keep blood sugar stabilized by balancing food intake. So, if someone is eating too many carbohydrate-rich foods and not enough fats or proteins, they may have a spike in blood sugar, which signals the body to accumulate fat, thus nullifying all best intentions.

1.9 IF ENABLES CELL REPAIR AND HELPS AVOID DISEASES

With IF you're literally giving your body and cells a chance to heal from stress and toxins. "By healing, your cells' mitochondria, lead to healthier cells and therefore better disease control," explains Galvin, "and letting the body repair itself naturally is also very beneficial for brain health." Although on mice, some studies have shown that fasting reduces age-related cognitive decline by disrupting the aging process, caused by genetics and behavior disease.

Mitochondria help transform the food we consume into energy, so when they weaken, they are vulnerable to mutations. "Because mitochondrial DNA has a limited ability to repair itself when damaged, they tend to develop over time," according to a report reported in Genetics Home Research, part of MedlinePlus. And he goes on to assert that "An accumulation of somatic mutations in mitochondrial DNA has been correlated with some types of cancer and with an elevated risk of some age-related diseases such as heart disease, Alzheimer's disease, and Parkinson's. Additionally, evidence indicates that the gradual accumulation of these mutations over a person's life may play a role in the natural stage of aging. According to the findings, helping your body fast is one way to reduce the risk of cancer and slow down the aging process."

2

Intermittent Fasting—
Types and benefits

2.1 TYPES OF INTERMITTENT FASTING

The first step you need to take is to establish a meal plan that suits your tastes and needs. Nutritionists have established several types of diets for IF that you have probably heard of by now. Almost all of them turn out to be very effective; you just have to decide which one is right for you.

2.1.1 DAILY INTERMITTENT FASTING

14:10

This is the most effective program for women. You can eat from 10:00 and fast from 20:00 to 10:00 the next day. But if you cannot survive without breakfast, this plan is not for you.

However, you could limit your breakfast to a cup of black tea or coffee until 10 am and not have dinner after 8 pm. However, some organization is required to make the mechanism work perfectly. Eating before 8 pm will lead you to go to bed a little earlier than usual, thus triggering a virtuous circle of greater well-being.

) THE 14:10 DIET

	DAY 1	DAY 2	DAY 3	DAY 4	DAY 5	DAY 6	DAY 7
MIDNIGHT / 4 AM	FAST	FAST	FAST	FAST	FAST	FAST	FAST
10 AM / 12 PM	First meal	First meal	First meal	First meal	First meal	First meal	First meal
4 PM	Last meal by 8PM	Last meal by 8PM	Last meal by 8PM	Last meal by 8PM	Last meal by 8PM	Last meal by 8PM	Last meal by 8PM
8 PM / MIDNIGHT	FAST	FAST	FAST	FAST	FAST	FAST	FAST

16:8

To follow this plan, also called the lean gains method, you should consume whatever you like within an 8-hour feeding window and fast for the remaining 16 hours. Who get the best results from this diet are men.

Typically, the time of fasting coincides with the time that passes between the evening meal, always before 8 pm, and the first meal of the day around lunchtime, thus skipping breakfast.

This plan would be even more effective if you have all meals between 11 am and 7 pm. During the remaining hours of the day, you can only consume unsweetened drinks, such as water, tea, and coffee. If you are wondering how many times per week to repeat this schedule, I will answer by telling you that this plan is a fasting regimen and that you should do it every day to see the results you have set for yourself. Remember that, even if I often use this term too, the IF it is not a diet, but a food routine that must become part of your lifestyle.

THE 16/8 METHOD

	DAY 1	DAY 2	DAY 3	DAY 4	DAY 5	DAY 6	DAY 7
Midnight							
4 AM	FAST	FAST	FAST	FAST	FAST	FAST	FAST
8 AM							
12 PM	First meal	First meal	First meal	First meal	First meal	First meal	First meal
4 PM	Last meal by 8pm	Last meal by 8pm	Last meal by 8pm	Last meal by 8pm	Last meal by 8pm	Last meal by 8pm	Last meal by 8pm
8 PM							
Midnight	FAST	FAST	FAST	FAST	FAST	FAST	FAST

20:4

This version of IF requires 4 hours of feeding and 20 hours of fasting. The choice of the moment of the day in which to eat is indifferent, once again it depends a lot on your lifestyle and your personal habits.

You will eat your meals around 2 pm and 6 pm every day and fast for the remaining 20 hours. This way, you'll have one or two simple meals in your 4-hour feeding interval.

With little time available, it is important to select the right foods, which provide the right energy. You can therefore prefer unsaturated fats and proteins by consuming adequate amounts of meat, fish, eggs, and vegetables. Outside the window, none of this.

2.1.2 Alternate Day Intermittent Fasting

This plan requires longer fasting times. In particular, this approach involves a normal day, during which we will behave as if nothing had happened, so 3 meals, and a complete day of fasting limiting the calorie intake by up to 75%.

On the fasting day, a maximum of 500 calories is allowed, precisely to allow you to follow the diet with less difficulty, without compromising its benefits.

Here too, there are no food restrictions but given the reduced calorie intake, it is better to focus on foods that allow you to increase the sense of satiety.

2.1.3 Weekly Intermittent Fasting

If you are a newbie to IF, this approach is definitely the simplest for you. This technique is not as successful as frequent intermittent fasting, however, many benefits can still be reaped. The concept is very simple.

Typically, people adapt quickly to this method for 24 hours and only eat once a day. This approach can be used 2–3 times a week; you can start your fasting period in the afternoon hours on Friday and have your first meal at noon on Sunday.

As a result, you skip about 2–3 meals a week, but beware that this approach won't help you lose weight.

2.1.4 EAT-STOP-EAT

5:2

The main premise of this diet strategy is that you have five days of daily consumption and two days of fasting. In reality, as with the alternate day regimen seen above, in the 2 days of fasting, you eat very little, no more than 500 calories, while on the other days you are free to eat what you want.

Just make sure your diet is as balanced as ever and contains protein, salad, fruit, and high-fiber foods. Be careful never to try to fast for two days in a row because, in addition to being unhealthy, you will not be successful. You absolutely have to divide the 2 days of fasting!

THE 5:2 DIET

DAY 1	DAY 2	DAY 3	DAY 4	DAY 5	DAY 6	DAY 7
Eats normally	Women: 500 calories Men: 600 calories	Eats normally	Eats normally	Women: 500 calories Men: 600 calories	Eats normally	Eats normally

2.1.5 Spontaneous meal skipping

Also called Random Intermittent Fasting. It is not necessary to follow a strict IF to see the first improvements, because another choice you can make is to skip meals from time to time, for example when you are not hungry or too distracted to prepare food.

One mistake people make is that they think they never have to skip meals to avoid putting their bodies into a fasting state. Your body can handle long periods of hunger, let alone skip a meal or two from time to time.

So if you are not hungry, skip breakfast and just eat a good lunch and dinner. Or, if you travel somewhere and can't find something you want to consume, do a little fast. Skipping a meal or two when you feel tempted to do so is certainly an excellent opportunity for your well-being.

SPONTANEOUS MEAL SKIPPING

DAY 1	DAY 2	DAY 3	DAY 4	DAY 5	DAY 6	DAY 7
Breakfast	Skipped Meal	Breakfast	Breakfast	Breakfast	Breakfast	Breakfast
Lunch	Lunch	Lunch	Lunch	Lunch	Lunch	Lunch
Dinner	Dinner	Dinner	Dinner	Skipped Meal	Dinner	Dinner

2.1.6   The warrior diet

Here, you fast during the day and eat at night within a 4-hour feeding window. Ori Hofmekler, a fitness expert, popularized this diet. It is a path that allows you to eliminate toxins and dispose of extra pounds through a diet made up of 2 daily phases: under-nutrition and over-nutrition.

According to Ori Hofmekler, alternating these phases and adopting an active lifestyle promotes vigor and strength, physical and mental, and keeps the metabolism alive. The under-feeding period is dedicated to purifying the body by limiting the energy intake by drinking plenty of water and/or detoxifying and diuretic centrifuged.

When you are in the period of over-feeding, you can eat until you are satisfied by always looking for a good balance of foods by favoring foods of different food groups and high protein.

THE WARRIOR DIET

	DAY 1	DAY 2	DAY 3	DAY 4	DAY 5	DAY 6	DAY 7
Midnight							
4 AM	Eating only small amounts of vegetables and fruits	Eating only small amounts of vegetables and fruits	Eating only small amounts of vegetables and fruits	Eating only small amounts of vegetables and fruits	Eating only small amounts of vegetables and fruits	Eating only small amounts of vegetables and fruits	Eating only small amounts of vegetables and fruits
8 AM							
12 PM							
4 PM	Large meal	Large meal	Large meal	Large meal	Large meal	Large meal	Large meal
8 PM							
Midnight							

2.1.7 Night fasting

As the name indicates, you will fast for 12 hours at night, in order to speed up your metabolism while respecting the biological clock.

It is also called autophagy fasting due to the 12-hour cycle, which mainly benefits our body by giving it time to eliminate excess toxins.

A great advantage of this form of fasting is that it is quick and easy to undertake, its secret lies in changing the time of the two main meals by postponing breakfast and anticipating dinner.

2.2 THE BEST FOODS TO EAT DURING INTERMITTENT FASTING

First, let's take a step back and review the basics: What benefits does your health derive from an IF diet?

You read a few pages ago that anti-aging effects are mainly attributed to better insulin regulation and that weight reduction is linked to reduced overall calorie consumption due to the so-called shorter feeding window.

Simply, because you have less time to eat throughout the day, you eat less. But a central concept, as in any diet, is to evaluate its feasibility in relation to your lifestyle. There are many great foods you MUST use to create your ultimate guide to IF and avoid nutritional deficiencies. Let's see them together.

2.2.1. Water

One of the most critical aspects of maintaining a balanced eating habit during IF is keeping the body hydrated. Our body's preferred energy supply is sugar stored in the liver, also known as glycogen. If this energy is burned, a huge amount of fluid and electrolytes disappear.

Since we run out of energy for 12–16 hours, at least eight glasses of water a day is a must, because it can reduce dehydration and also lead to an improvement in blood flow, memory, and muscle and joint strength during the IF regimen.

2.2.2 Lentils

This healthy legume offers high fiber potency with 32% of the total fiber requirement satisfied in just half a cup. In addition to this, lentils provide a good source of iron (about 15% of the daily requirement).

Another very important nutrient, especially for active women who are following IF.

2.2.3 Unrefined grains

Carbohydrates are an important aspect of life and most likely aren't the threat when it comes to weight loss. Since a good portion of your day would be spent fasting during this diet, it is vital to think carefully about how to get enough calories without going overboard.

Conversely, a balanced diet minimizes refined foods. There will be a time and a place for things like wholemeal bread, crackers, and cookies as these foods are more easily digested for a trained physique. For this reason, if you plan on exercising or training frequently during your D.I., this can be a particularly good source of energy on the go.

2.2.4 Hummus

One of the softest and tastiest snacks known to mankind. Hummus is another extraordinary vegetable protein and a perfect way to increase the nutritional value of classic dishes such as sandwiches: try replacing it with mayonnaise. If you're brave enough to make your own hummus, don't forget that the trick to the best recipe is tahini and garlic.

2.2.5 Potatoes

Comparable to bread, white potatoes are metabolized with minimal effort by the body. And when combined with a protein source, they are a great post-workout snack to recharge hungry muscles.

Another advantage is that once cold, potatoes form a resistant starch, perfect for feeding the beneficial bacteria in the gut.

2.2.6 Smoothies

If you don't want to use a daily supplement, consider getting a double dose of vitamins by making organic fruit and vegetable-filled smoothies. They are a perfect way to ingest several different foods, with several essential nutrients.

2.2.7 Blueberries

Don't be confused by their miniature appearance: blueberries are proof that good things come in small packages too! Studies have found that antioxidants are essential for the survival and youthfulness of the physique. Blueberries are a perfect source of antioxidants, which help detoxify the body of free radicals and avoid widespread cell damage.

2.2.8 Stronger milk with vitamin D

The recommended calcium intake for an adult is 1,000 milligrams per day, exactly what you would get from drinking three cups of milk per day.

With a narrow feeding window, the chances of consuming so much calcium are very slim, so you need to choose foods rich in it. Milk enriched with vitamin D increases the body's processing of calcium, which can help keep bones healthy.

To increase your regular calcium intake, you can add milk to sweets or cereals or simply consume it with meals. If you're not a fan of drinks, calcium-rich but non-dairy options include tofu and soy products, as well as leafy greens like kale.

2.2.9 Clarified butter

A drizzle of olive oil has tremendous health benefits, but there are many other varieties of oil you can use. If you don't want to heat the oil above the smoke point, try using clarified butter instead of olive oil.

Basically, clarified butter has a much higher smoke point which makes it lighter than oil.

2.2.10 Papaya

In the last few hours of your IF you may experience hunger symptoms, particularly if you are just starting out with it. This fruit will potentially help fill you up without making you feel tired and irritable. Papaya produces a particular enzyme called papain, which works to break down proteins. Taking this tropical fruit in a protein-rich meal will help its absorption and reduce swelling.

2.2.11 Branched-chain amino acids (BCAA)

BCAAs are a great muscles building aid for athletes who like fast or vigorous cardio workouts as their first activity in the morning. They can also be consumed at any time of the day (fasting or not) to prevent catabolism and preserve lean muscle mass. If you have chosen to follow a vegan diet, be careful, because this product is mostly composed of duck feathers.

Well, are you convinced now? Do you want to start your IF journey in a simple, fun, and healthy way? Here is a plan that will guide you day by day with the directions to take.

Enjoy your journey!!

2.3.1 DAY 1

Today's Task: 12 hours of fasting

Today's Mission: Choose your IF program

During the first week, I suggest you start progressively with the IF. For example, start the first day with a 12-hour fast and increase by one hour a day to 16 hours on day 5. It is safer for the body and brain to get used to various diet programs in this way.

It would also be advisable for you to select a plan that matches your lifestyle for real, and that you can follow for a full 21-day period, starting today.

As with all things, consistency is one of the most important elements that lead to success.

2.3.2 DAY 2

Today's Task: 13 hours of fasting

Today's Mission: Learn the basics of IF

Today the fasting period is increased by 1 hour, therefore 13 hours without eating. On this second day, it's important that you focus on some healthy eating habits that can help you reach your goals: for example, start with the consumption of whole foods and avoid fats, processed foods, and empty carbohydrates.

In the last part of this book, there are some foods and recipes that you can cook and consume for the best results. In general, think of simple but delicious and nutritious meals that you can make at home, such as poached eggs with spinach, meatballs, and zucchini, feta salad, or homemade hummus for a snack.

2.3.3 DAY 3

Today's Task: 14 hours of fasting

Today's Mission: Define your rewards

When you start developing a new habit, like a new diet lifestyle, rewards are important. So, for day 3, it's time for you to determine what your reward will be for each successful day.

Why is this step so important? A reward sends a constructive signal to the brain, like "Doing this is good. We should do it more!" and it is something that makes you feel good.

Ideally, the right benefit when you reach a goal related to your fasting plan should be related to your basic needs for relaxation, socialization, food, or play.

The reward can also be quick but powerful, for example, it can simply be a gesture of victory you do right after you reach a goal, like cheering yourself up and saying "Good job" or ticking off another day of IF successfully completed.

Or you can pursue a symbolic strategy: for example, for each success achieved, you receive 1 token. When you've earned 5 tokens, you treat yourself to the real reward and spend an evening at your favorite restaurant.

2.3.4 DAY 4

Today's Task: 15 hours of fasting

Today's Mission: Make a protein-rich lunch!

Your body needs it today, after 15 hours of fasting. To recover, eat a high-protein snack that will help you reach your weight loss goal.

For example, you can prepare vegetables with a dish of your choice, such as meat, fish, legumes, beans, eggs, tofu, almonds, grilled beef, or seeds. If you are looking for some recipes, I suggest you try a refreshing summer salad of pomegranate with wild salmon: delicious!

2.3.5 DAY 5

Today's Task: 16 hours of fasting

Today's Mission: when you're hungry, drink black coffee or water

On the fifth day of the plan, you will reach the so-called "cruising speed" of 16/8, which means that you will fast for 16 hours and feed for 8.

I assure you it will be relatively simple to do. I have already experienced it as well as hundreds of people who have successfully faced the 21-day challenge.

If you can't reach the 16 hours of fasting and quenching your hunger, we recommend consuming black coffee. It's packed with antioxidants that will help you lose weight, but don't overdo it!

Keep in mind that the coffee we are speaking about is dark. This means no sugar, no syrup or creams, no cappuccino or milk, just black coffee. If you want to add something tasty, use organic stevia sweetener, but be careful as it can trigger hunger.

If you are not a coffee drinker, you can replace it with a cup of green or black tea, or simply a glass of water. I assure you that sometimes the feeling of hunger disappears after drinking just a couple of glasses of water.

2.3.6 DAY 6

Today's Task: 16 hours of fasting

Today's Mission: Go for a walk

Is it your goal to lose weight during these 21 days of fasting? It is important to follow a well-balanced diet and we recommend that you get some exercise in your daily routine. Just before you break your fast, go for a walk. Even a short 20-minute walk will be enough.

Walking is a great way to improve your fitness, your mood, and actually get some fresh air. Above all, taking a walk will distract you from your appetite and make the last few hours of fasting smoother.

2.3.7 DAY 7

Today's Task: 16 hours of fasting

Today's Mission: Go for a walk

Keep the goal of the previous day and focus on the goals achieved during your week of fasting. Taking a full-body image, recording the weight, and comparing it are part of the transformation process.

You may begin to see the first signs of weight loss and/or a change in your physical appearance. Also, I'd like you to take a second to reflect on your success. How do you feel? Do you feel changed? Do you have more energy? More resistance? Has your attitude changed? Or your skin? And so on.

This exercise will help you recognize when and, more importantly, why you may be having difficulty. This will help you take steps to speed up your results by making the IF a new sustainable habit.

2.4 WHAT TO EAT FOR BREAKFAST?

It is always best to come out of your fasting state slowly. In order not to overload the digestive tract too much, I recommend that you take small amounts of more easily digestible foods.

Breaking your fast with foods high in calories, sugar, or even fiber can be very exhausting for your body, because they can be hard to digest, thus causing bloating and discomfort. So I recommend: no smelly cheeseburgers, cakes, or fizzy drinks. And no fresh foods, fiber-rich nuts, and seeds, these can also be hard to digest.

On the other hand, foods rich in nutrients that are easy to absorb and with a small amount of protein and good fats will help you break your fast easily.

Below you will find some examples of what to eat to break your fast.

2.4.1 Smoothies

Blended drinks can be a gentler way to introduce nutrients into your body as they contain less fiber than whole, raw fruits, and vegetables.

2.4.2 Soups

Soups of easily digestible proteins and carbohydrates, such as lentils, tofu, or pasta, can gently break your fast. Avoid soups made with cream or with a large number of raw vegetables rich in fiber.

2.4.3 Dried fruit

Dates are a concentrated source of nutrients, frequently used for breakfasts in Saudi Arabia. Apricots and raisins can have similar effects.

2.4.4 Fermented foods

Try sugar-free yogurt or kefir. Breaking the fast with healthy foods that can be better tolerated can help replenish important nutrients and electrolytes and facilitate the return of so-called "normal" food to your diet.

2.4.5 Healthy fats

Foods like eggs or avocados can be great first foods to eat after vegetables. Cooked, soft, and starchy vegetables like potatoes are also good options.

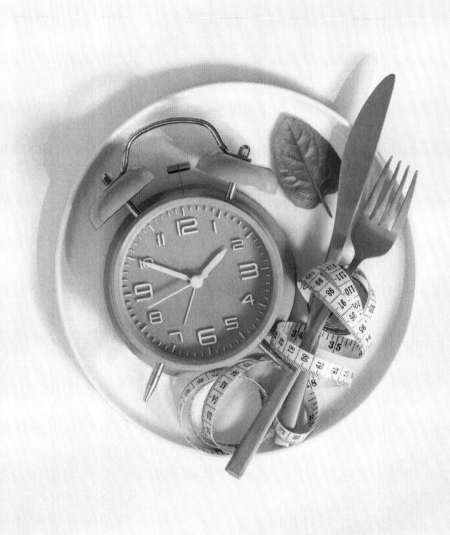

3

Pros and cons of intermittent fasting

As you have already learned, there are different types of IF, ranging from complete banning of food on certain days of the week to limited intervals of the day. These different habits of life allow to reach and support a stable weight and to have a better physical shape even among already balanced individuals. Let's see what are IF's pros and cons.

3.1 PROS

3.1.1 Easy to follow

Dietary preferences often depend on the consumption of specific products and the limitation or exclusion of others. Learning the basic rules of an eating style saves a lot of time. For example, there are entire books devoted to understanding the Dash diet or discovering how to run a Mediterranean food program. In a diet plan that involves prolonged fasting, you actually feed yourself based on the time or day of the week. If you have decided which IF method it's best for you, all you need is a clock or a calendar to know what to eat.

3.1.2 No macronutrient limitations

Macronutrients are important ingredients that must be introduced in large quantities, as they represent the most important energy source for the body. Carbohydrates, fats, and proteins belong to this category. There are common food plans that severely limit these macronutrients.

For example, many people adopt a low-carb diet to improve fitness or lose weight. Others, a low-fat diet for health reasons. Each of these plans allows you to follow a different eating style, sometimes changing your favorite dishes with new and potentially unknown ones.

This leads you to learn about new recipes and buy new types of foods, which is certainly not a bad thing, but during intermittent fasting, you will not have to go through any of this, simply because nothing is limited or prohibited.

3.1.3 It could potentially increase longevity

One of the most cited effects of IF is longevity. According to the National Institute on Aging, rodent experiments show that when mice are placed in programs that heavily limit calories (often during fasting periods), there is an average lengthening of lifespan along with a reduction in mortality, due to some diseases, in particular tumors.

Is it plausible to say that this benefit is also found in human beings? According to the experts, YES! Of course, many long-term studies are still needed on the subject in order to definitively dismiss the issue.

According to another study published in 2010, there was empirical evidence linking religious fasting to the effects of long-term longevity, but it was difficult to ascertain whether fasting was the cause or if other factors were responsible.

3.1.4 No calorie counts

People who are trying to achieve or maintain a healthier weight tend to stop counting calories. Although nutrition labels are readily available on many items, the task of calculating portion sizes and tabulating regular counts manually or on a mobile app can be tedious.

Some research published in 2011 showed that people are more inclined to adopt plans when all pre-measured calorie-controlled meals are delivered. Commercial diets like WW, Jenny Craig, and others offer these programs for a fee, but families often don't have the money to pay for these types of services, especially in the long run.

IF offers a convenient option, because just a little calorie count is required. In some cases, calorie restriction (and consequently weight loss) occurs when food is removed or significantly reduced on certain days or at certain times of the day.

3.1.5 Promotes weight loss

I don't want to dwell too much on this topic; I have already dealt with it a few pages back. In an important meta-analysis conducted in 2018, scientists compared the results of 11 different studies lasting 8–24 weeks, highlighting that both IF that constant energy restriction achieved similar results when weight loss and metabolic changes were the goals.

In the same context, they also discovered that in some situations the results of weight loss may depend on age. They investigated the impact of intermittent fasting on young men aged 20 and over 50. The result was that IF reduced body mass in younger men, but not in older men, not altering muscle strength in either group.

3.1.6 Eating without restriction

Anyone who has ever tried a diet to obtain a medical benefit, such as a healthier weight, knows perfectly well how much they tend to crave the so-called "forbidden foods." A report released in 2017 concluded that the harder you are to stick to a strict diet, the more likely you are to fail at weight loss.

It is considerably easier to follow an IF program. Food deprivation only applies during these limited hours, and on the non-fasting hours or days of the plan, you can usually consume whatever you want. I recommend you to call the NON-fasting days of your plan your "feast days."

Of course, consuming fatty foods is not the healthiest way to take advantage of IF, but limiting them on fasting days is also beneficial.

3.1.7 Glucose control

This eating pattern is able to help people with type 2 diabetes control their blood sugar through weight reduction for overweight or obese people, but it can also increase insulin sensitivity in healthy people.

In 2018, several studies showed the effectiveness of fasting (accompanied by medical monitoring and 6-hour dietary training) in reversing insulin resistance while maintaining regulation of their blood sugars for a 7-month cycle. In all three scenarios, patients were able to end insulin treatment, lose weight, lower belly size, and see an overall rise in blood sugar.

3.1.8 Other health benefits

Some findings have linked IF with a number of other health benefits. However, almost all scholars agree that further study is needed to adequately appreciate its value. For example, in 2018, researchers reported that fasting during Ramadan contributes to a reduction in total LDL (the "bad" cholesterol), triglycerides, and at the same time an improvement in HDL levels (the "good" cholesterol).

Another 2014 study showed that IF could be an efficient approach to addressing low-grade systemic inflammation and some chronic diseases related to age and immune function without losing physical performance.

3.2 CONS

Studies exploring IF implications often refer to some negative effects that can arise during the fasting phase of the routine. For example, it isn't unusual to feel a bad mood, suffer from heartburn, nausea, sleepiness, constipation, dehydration, decreased sleep quality, or anemia.

IF can be harmful to those with asthma, elevated LDL cholesterol levels, exaggeratedly high amounts of uric acid in the blood, cardiovascular disease, hyperglycemia, and liver and kidney disorders.

3.2.1 Reduced physical activity

One of the major consequences of IF can be a lack of exercise. Its various types give indications on when not to eat, but don't provide guidelines relating to physical exercise. In fact, those who follow it can feel so exhausted that they struggle to reach their daily goals and can even change their normal training habits. I recommend that you evaluate day by day how the IF affects your physical activity sessions.

3.2.2 Medications

Many patients who take medicines find that taking them with meals tends to alleviate the side effects. Some prescriptions clearly suggest taking them with food. Therefore, taking medication while fasting can be a problem. Anyone who needs to take medications should speak to his doctor before starting any path of IF, to make sure that the fasting phase doesn't interact with the efficacy or side effects of the drug.

3.2.3 Huge hunger

It's normal for those who are in the fasting phase of an IF food routine to feel extreme hunger, which can become more intense when surrounded by people who don't follow any particular diet and therefore eat normal snacks and meals. A good piece of advice is to take this path with your partner or a trusted friend. Anyway, it's very important to always keep this sentence in mind: "Hold on and don't give up!"

3.2.4 It can promote overeating

During the feeding state, the amount of food and the duration of the meal are not limited. As a result, some people may indulge in an "ad libitum" meal, overeating. For example, if you feel hungry after a full day of fasting, you may be tempted to overeat, or worse, eat the wrong foods.

3.2.5 No focus on healthy foods

The key to any strategy in this diet is rhythm, not food choice. Therefore, there are no restrictions, and foods that offer good nutrition are not "encouraging." For this reason, those who adopt any IF plan may not be able to consume a balanced diet. Without good help, you may not be able to cook healthy, with healthy oils, or prefer vegetables and select whole grains over processed grains. So, be very careful!

3.2.6 Long-term limitations

While the practice of intermittent fasting is not new, much of the research studying its benefits have only recently been discovered. As a result, it is not yet known precisely whether the benefits will last in the long term.

For now, the safest course of action is to consult with your doctor when choosing to start an IF plan, to track the results together and any benefits or problems that will arise, to ensure the healthiest eating style for you and your body.

3.3. COMMON MYTHS ABOUT INTERMITTENT FASTING

If you are practicing IF or thinking about doing it, it is essential to learn the right information to be able to start on the right foot and enjoy the benefits of weight loss and the increased energy you will feel. Unfortunately, there is a lot of misinformation about it. I bet you've probably already read things like:

- Fasting slows down metabolism,

- It's not good to drink water during a fast,

- Fasting shrivels the muscles.

These fasting theories aren't true, they are based on rumors, conjectures, and false myths. Let's see them one by one:

Myth No. 1: Fasting slows down your metabolism

Some people worry that fasting reduces the resting metabolic rate, meaning it burns fewer calories. The widespread fear is that you can gain weight like a three-toed sloth once you quit this diet. This is what occurs in calorie restriction diets, which means consuming 50% to 85%

of the calories the body consumes regularly, over the long term. Your body adapts to the reduced energy consumption without changing for years.

If you have ever watched The Biggest Loser TV show, you will surely have noticed the calorie reduction that patients/competitors are subjected to. They lose weight and frequently regain it, but the fans of the program never or almost never talk about this aspect.

Does the Yo-Yo effect also occur for the IF? NO. In a study done in 2005, conducted in the American Journal of Clinical Nutrition, overweight people who observed alternate day fasting maintained a regular metabolic rate for most of the three weeks, while also burning more fat.

Myth No. 2: It's not good to drink water during a fast

Some religious fasts, including Ramadan, require both food and water restrictions. Unfortunately, since fasting has a diuretic impact, limiting water can contribute to dangerous dehydration. That is why doctors pay special attention to fluid consumption when supervising patients undertaking clinical fasts.

Myth No. 3: Fasting shrivels the muscles

Fasting doesn't seem like the right way to build muscles. But don't you keep making protein shakes? Okay, you definitely need nutrition, but you don't need it 24/7.

It was shown in 2019 that some women undergoing an IF 16:8 regimen gained the same amount of muscle and power as women following a traditional diet. Here's the problem: your body works hard to maintain muscle in times of energy shortage. During those times you consume body fat (not muscle) for energy needs.

Myth No. 4: Fasting makes you eat more

After a fast, you will be hungry! A lot of people think that the appetite in the final stage of the fasted state fuels the need and desire for food. Data, however, don't support this concern: most fasting studies encourage patients to consume as much as they want.

They eat their fill and continue to lose weight. You will find that you will consume less food, not more, in any type of IF. This moderate calorie restriction, in particular, promotes a slight weight reduction without slowing down the metabolism.

Myth No. 5: It's for everyone

IF is trendy and everyone is talking about it. Many are already following it and others are starting just as you are reading this book. Attention, although fasting is safe and nutritious for most people, it is not suitable for everyone, indeed it should be avoided for:

- Pregnant and breastfeeding women

- Children

- People suffering from eating disorders

- People with thyroid disorders

- People suffering from diseases related to insulin levels.

Groups of people listed above must eat more food than they need, not less. The possibility of nutritional loss outweighs the possible benefits of fasting.

Many slightly overweight people who experience elevated blood sugar levels may undertake IF, but with caution. Before doing so, however, I recommend once again consulting your trusted doctor/dietician, because although fasting can be therapeutic, medical assistance is necessary to avoid the onset of hypoglycemia (dangerously low blood sugar levels).

Myth No. 6: Fasting drains your energy

If food is fuel, don't energy levels plummet without it?

In the end, of course! But as you fast intermittently, your cells tap into an alternative energy source—body fat—and there's plenty of it to make it through the day. A lean individual (for example 70 kg with 10% body fat) has incredible fat reserves to meet energy needs during fasting. If you do the math, 7kg of fat equals over 60,000 calories of energy!

All those who undertake the IF report feeling very good and full of energy. It makes sense, as blood is drawn from the tissues and digestive organs during a large meal.

Myth No. 7: You cannot concentrate while fasting

Think back to when you were fiercely hungry. It wasn't your most Zen moment. When you start following a daily practice of prolonged fasting, you will no longer feel this way. When cells start using body fat for fuel, appetite hormones stabilize.

When you burn body fat, you release ketones, small molecules that feed the brain with pure, usable energy. For this reason, entering ketosis increases concentration, memory, and emphasis in the elderly.

4

Intermittent Fasting and Training

Exercise is a must, not only for those who follow any type of diet but in general as a lifestyle. Following this diet and continuing to carry out the correct training is perhaps a little more complicated.

So here are eight things you need to know to train safely and effectively while fasting.

4.1 THINGS TO KNOW ABOUT INTERMITTENT FASTING AND TO WORK ON

4.1.1 Keep exercising while fasting. But relax!

Fasting exercises have their advantages. Exercising with an empty stomach can help with weight loss because your body would draw on stored energy reserves in the form of glycogen and fat instead of burning your most recent meal. When you train on an empty stomach, however, there is a risk that your body will start attacking the muscles for energy. This is because high-intensity exercises need a lot of carbohydrates for fuel.

This means that running fast or doing your daily Crossfit exercise while fasting, or at the end of your fast, can greatly reduce the benefits of your workout. You may not even have enough energy to train if you are new to this diet.

An excellent alternative to high-intensity physical exercises, which certainly cause negative effects when fasted, is low-intensity cardio because it works mainly on fats. Exercises suitable for cardio include cycling, jogging, meditation, swimming, and gentle Pilates.

4.1.2 Listen to your body

If you have certain health conditions (especially those that can trigger dizziness, including low blood sugar or low blood pressure), exercise when you're not fasting. Pay attention to your body and do what makes you feel good! If you feel weak while exercising, rest, gather energy and hydrate before moving on to the fasting phase or before moving your training into this phase.

4.1.3 Start adapt yourself to a fat-burning metabolism

It takes a couple of weeks for your body to respond to any changes or new habits, so adopt a low-carb lifestyle before fasting to give your body time to adjust. If you experience chronic fatigue, weakness, dizziness, depression, burnout, nausea, or find yourself recovering from your workouts very slowly, it's time to slow down.

IF and exercise can be complicated and daunting to manage at the same time. Warning: extra workouts can make you feel hungrier in general, which can make fasting much more challenging, particularly if the intensity of these exercises is too strong.

4.1.4 Hydration

It is essential to drink plenty of water and supplements while fasting, especially when you fast and exercise at the same time. If electrolytes are not controlled properly, headaches, hypoglycemia, nausea, dizziness, low blood pressure, and cramps can occur.

Replenish your electrolytes with organic coconut water, supplement capsules, or zero-calorie electrolyte drinks. Avoid sports drinks that are high in calories, caffeine, and other diuretics. Make sure you are eating enough sodium and potassium as well as being adequately hydrated.

4.1.5 Refuel after a workout

Improve your fast during your feeding window by consuming sufficient amounts of protein, high-fiber carbohydrates, and balanced fats. Follow your high-intensity exercise and get protein within 30 minutes of completing your workout. If you're doing moderate-intensity cardio on an empty stomach, train at the end of your fasting period so you can refuel soon after. Go for entirely organic foods that balance proteins and carbohydrates. For example, scrambled eggs with vegetables, or if you're on the go and need a quick and easy post-workout feeding solution, consider a protein bar or protein shake.

4.1.6 Time of day when you prefer to train

If you use to work out before 8 am, you may need to change your feeding schedule so that you can eat right after an aerobic exercise. If you are a lover of afternoon workouts, this is a great time to do some weight lifting. However, remember that low-intensity exercises can be performed at any time of the day.

4.1.7 Vary your workouts

As the body continues to burn fat, combine high-intensity training and exercise to gain muscle mass. This will clearly support you in your IF plan as well. On days when you can do morning exercise, focus on cardio, while when you can hit the gym in the evening, exercise will be your best ally. On those days when you feel more drained, don't hesitate to take a break or experiment with meditation or Pilates.

4.1.8 Use mineral salts

Low-calorie drinks such as coconut water or natural sports drinks will help ensure that your body receives replenishment of minerals and supplements without breaking fast.

4.2. HOW TO CHOOSE THE RIGHT TRAINING FOR THE IF PLAN

Not all physical exercises are the same when it comes to doing them while fasting. Some forms of training are more demanding on the muscles and require a meal immediately afterward, others may require more carbohydrate consumption at the start of the day.

4.2.1 Cardio and HIIT

When done correctly, fasted cardio can be a perfect addition to your fitness routine. Depending on the type of exercise you perform, you may or not have a meal right after. If you're out for a slow, steady morning run, you may be fine for hours after you've finished exercising and then wait before eating again. But if this makes you feel faint and lightheaded, eat right after you stop exercising. You need to give your body time to adjust and be able to achieve these fasting conditions.

4.2.2 Yoga, barre, and low-intensity workouts

On days when you feel low on energy, even and especially during the initial period of the plan, the best exercises for your body are the low-intensity ones, both in the fasting phase and in the feeding phase. As for the IF plans, the exercises indicated are barre, Pilates, and meditation and can be safely performed during the fasting window because, as I wrote previously, they're not the high intensity and so they do not overload the body by sending it into an energy deficit. With this type of exercise, you will find that there is no need to replenish once the workout is over, as with high-intensity exercises.

4.2.3 High-intensity training

If you want to gain muscle mass, you need to get refined proteins and carbohydrates before and after training. If you are working on your body to improve mass and endurance, then you should ideally train just before breaking the fast, not towards the end of your feeding window, when you can no longer replenish your energy. To make your muscles work well and achieve the weight lifting or HIIT exercise goals you have set for yourself, it is recommended that you consume some calories before starting training.

This will allow your body to have the momentum you need, but even then it all comes down to what makes you feel better. You have to experiment and balance! "What are my fitness goals? How do I feel during training?" If you realize that you are completely exhausted and therefore cannot train successfully, something is wrong. Stop for a second and collect your ideas.

4.3. PROGRAM TO GET THE MOST OUT OF FASTING AND TRAINING

This program depends on your specific fasting needs and can be adjusted to what you think works better for you:

- Monday: cardio followed by a high-protein breakfast.

- Tuesday: complex carbohydrate lunch (pasta, rice, or potatoes), and in the afternoon high-intensity workout followed by dinner.

- Wednesday: yoga, barre, pilates, or other low-intensity workouts.

- Thursday: cardio followed by a high-protein breakfast.

- Friday: complex carbohydrate lunch, and in the afternoon high-intensity workout followed by dinner.

- Saturday or Sunday: yoga, barre, pilates, or other low-intensity workouts.

4.4.1 Starting drastically with IF

Starting suddenly with the IF is one of the biggest mistakes you can make. If you start without the right preparation, you will almost certainly face a catastrophe. Going from having three regular meals or 6 smaller meals a day to eating within four hours is definitely a difficult change for your body.

Instead, do this: slow down your meals gradually and slowly embrace fasting. If you're opting for the 16:8 process, progressively extend the hours between meals so you can easily fit into a 16-hour time frame.

4.4.2 Not choosing the right plan for IF

You can decide which plan to take and buy whole grains, fish, poultry, fruits, vegetables, and nutritious side dishes like quinoa and legumes. But if you haven't selected the fasting strategy that best suits your body and lifestyle, you won't have the success you deserve. If you are a passionate and frequent gym 6 days a week, absolute fasting for two of those days may not be the perfect plan. So rather than starting a plan without thinking about it, evaluate your lifestyle first and choose the plan that best fits your routine and behavior.

4.4.3 Eating too much in your feeding window

One of the reasons people want to try IF is the belief that the little time they spend eating makes them consume fewer calories than they should. But this does not happen! Even once the IF has started, it is not uncommon to see the intake of the normal amount of calories, with the result of not being able to lose weight and not achieve the benefits of this diet. So even if what you are about to read seems obvious, be sure not to consume your regular 2000 calorie amount during your feeding window.

Rather, commit to eating 1200 to 1500 calories during the time period from breakfast to your last meal of the day. Many meals you eat will depend on how long your feeding window lasts, whether it's 4, 6, or 8 hours. If you really need to eat more and are in a state of deprivation, think about varying the program you have decided to follow, or loosen your fast for a day to refocus yourself. You will be back on track very easily!!

4.4.4 Eating the wrong foods in your feeding window

Another of the most common mistakes for those who undertake the IF, in addition to overeating, is the intake of "wrong foods." Again, it seems obvious that you will not feel well if you only eat unbalanced, fatty, or sugary foods during your diet. Instead, eat lean proteins, healthy fats, nuts, legumes, unrefined grains, and healthy fruits and vegetables.

Here are some tips that may be useful for a healthy diet when you are not fasting:

- Avoid processed foods, prefer whole foods

- Read nutrition labels and become familiar with banned ingredients, such as high fructose corn syrup and modified palm oil

- Cook and eat at home instead of at the restaurant;

- Balance your plate with fiber, carbohydrates, and healthy fats, and lean proteins

- Check your sodium intake and watch out for hidden sugars

4.4.5 Limiting calories in the fasting window

It is not healthy to eat fewer than 1200 calories during the day. Not only that, but it has the negative potential to slow down your metabolic rate resulting in you starting to lose muscle mass instead of increasing it if you don't run for cover right away.

4.4.6 Unknowingly breaking intermittent fasting

It is essential to be aware of the hidden fast switches. Did you realize that the taste of sugar also causes the brain to release insulin? And this release of insulin essentially breaks the fast. Here are some unexpected foods, supplements, and products that can break a fast and trigger an insulin response:

- Vitamins, like vitamins from gummy bears, contain sugar and fat

- Using toothpaste and mouthwash containing the xylitol sweetener

- Supplements that contain additives such as maltodextrins and pectins

- Some pain relievers may contain sugar in the coating.

Breaking the fast is a common mistake for those starting to practice IF. When you are not feeding, clean your teeth with a mixture of baking soda and water and read labels carefully before consuming vitamins and supplements.

4.4.7 Not drinking enough during the IF

This meal plan requires you to stay hydrated a lot. Keep in mind that the body does not absorb water that is normally absorbed with food. As a result, the side effects could make you sick. If you get dehydrated, you can experience headaches, muscle cramps, and extreme hunger. To avoid this mistake and suffer from the symptoms described above, remember during the day to take some of these liquids of your choice:

- Water

- Water and 1–2 tablespoons of apple cider vinegar (this could also curb hunger)

- Black coffee (be careful not to overdo it)

- Black, herbal, oolong, or green tea

4.4.8 Do not exercise during intermittent fasting

Some people believe that it would be better not to exercise during the fasting period, when in fact it is the perfect situation. Exercise makes you burn the accumulated fat in your body. Also, when you train, your growth hormone levels increase, thus aiding muscle growth. There are, however, some guidelines to follow to get the most out of your workouts.

To get the best results from your efforts, keep these points in mind:

- If the type of exercise is intense, eat first to be sure to make your glycogen stores available.

- Base your exercise on the fasting method; if you are fasting for 24 hours, do not plan an intensive activity that day.

- Time your workouts during feeding periods and then eat healthy carbohydrates and proteins within 30 minutes of exercising.

- Listen to your body's signals; if you feel faint or lightheaded, take a break or stop exercising.

- Stay hydrated while fasting and especially during training.

\4.4.9. Being too hard on yourself if you make any mistakes during IF

A fall does not imply failure! You will have days in which following this plan will be particularly difficult and you will think that you will not be able to keep up. It is perfectly normal to take a break if necessary. So if it happens, don't worry but give yourself a break and restart the next day, sticking to the balanced meal plan, but treat yourself to a surprise, like a fantastic protein shake or a healthy steak and broccoli to get you going with the right energy.

Don't let the IF take over your entire life. Consider it a part of your good routine and don't forget to take care of yourself in other ways as well. Enjoy a good read, exercise, spend more time with your friends, and live in the healthiest way possible. It's just part of the process of being the strongest version of yourself.

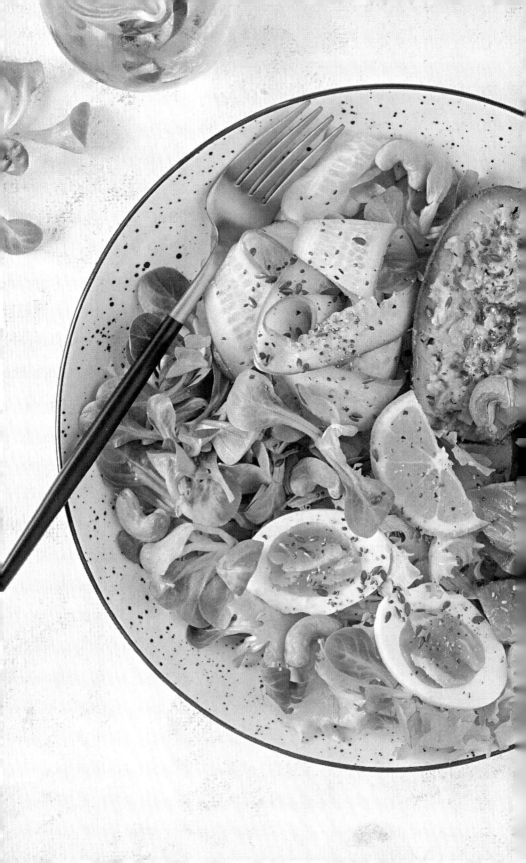

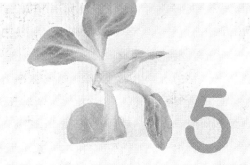

5

Recipes

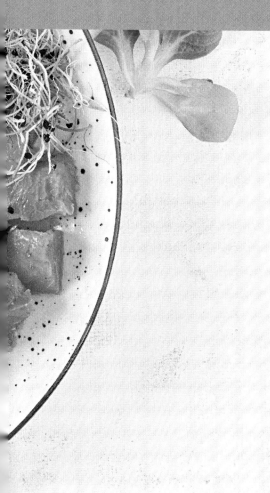

5.1. Mediterranean Salad with Sardines

Cooking Time:	Servings:	Difficulty:
15'	4	Easy

Ingredients:

3 oz. green leaves

5 chopped black olives

1 tbsp. desalted capers

2 cans sardines, drained

1 tbsp. olive oil

1 tbsp. red wine vinegar

1 glass tomato sauce

Directions:

1. Spread the green leaves into 4 plates.
2. Sprinkle the olives and capers.
3. Coarsely chop the sardines and add them to the salad.
4. Mix the tomato sauce with the oil and vinegar and toss over the salad.

5.2 Spiced Chicken and Pineapple Salad

Cooking Time:	Servings:	Difficulty:
10'	2	Easy

Ingredients:

1 red chili, deseeded and chopped

1 small red onion, halved and thinly sliced

1 tbsp. sweet chili sauce

2 tbsp. white wine vinegar

8 oz. pineapple juice

3 oz. bag leaf, mixed

5 oz. pack chicken breast, cooked and sliced

Handful cherry tomatoes, halved

Small bunch coriander, leaves picked

Directions:

1. Drain the pineapple juice and set it aside. Chop the rings into pieces if they're in rings. If serving as a snack, mix the chicken, onion, leaves, coriander, and tomatoes in a mixing bowl and split into 2 containers.

2. To make the dressing, mix 2 tsp. pineapple juice, red chili, vinegar, and sweet chili sauce in a shallow jam jar or lidded bottle with some seasoning, and before serving, toss with the salad.

5.3 Squash Salad and Beetroot with Horseradish Cream

Cooking Time:	Servings:	Difficulty:
45'	12	Medium

Ingredients:

6 red onions, sliced

4 tbsp. olive oil

2 tbsp. red wine vinegar

2 lb. raw beetroot, peeled and cut into 8 wedges

3 lb. large butternut squash (the long one) peeled and sliced without seeds

1 tbsp. soft brown sugar

For the Horseradish Cream

1 lemon juice

6 oz. sour cream

3 tbsp. horseradish cream

3 oz. watercress, large stems removed

Directions:

1. Preheat the oven to 390°F or 350°F.
2. Into a large baking sheet, pour the ingredients.
3. Mix the vinegar and sugar together until the sugar is completely dissolved, then add the oil.
4. Pour this dressing over the vegetables, stir and roast for 40–45 minutes, stirring halfway through cooking, until the pumpkins, onions, and beets are cooked and tender.
5. To make horseradish cream, mix horseradish, sour cream, lemon juice in a mixing bowl.
6. To serve, mix the roasted vegetables with the watercress in a large bowl or serving dish, then drizzle with the horseradish cream.
7. You can serve this dish either hot or cold.

5.4 Asian Chicken Salad

Cooking Time:	Servings:	Difficulty:
10'	2	Easy

Ingredients:

About 1 tbsp. Zest and juice of ½ lime

Large handful coriander, roughly chopped

3 ½ oz. bag salad leaves, mixed

1 tsp. caster sugar

1 tbsp. fish sauce

1 chicken breast, boneless, skinless

½ chili, deseeded and thinly sliced

¼ red onion

¼ cucumber, sliced lengthways

Directions:

1. Place the chicken in a pot of cold water, then bring to a boil and simmer for 10 minutes. Remove the meat from a pan and shred it. Stir the lime zest, fish sauce, juice, and sugar together until the sugar is dissolved.

2. In a container, mix the leaves and coriander, and then cover with the chicken, pepper, onion, and cucumber. Toss the salad with dressing in a different pan until preparing to serve.

5.5 Cobb Salad with Brown Derby Dressing

Cooking Time:	Servings:	Difficulty:
30'	2	Easy

Ingredients:

1/2 cup blue cheese, crumbled

tbsp. chives, chopped fine

hardboiled egg

1 avocado, sliced in half, seeded and peeled

1 bunch chicory lettuce

1/2 head romaine lettuce

1/2 lb. turkey breast, smoked

2 medium tomatoes, skinned and seeded

1/2 head iceberg lettuce

1/2 bunch watercress

Dressing

2 cloves garlic, minced very fine

2 tbsp. olive oil

1/8 tsp. Dijon mustard

1/2 tsp. black pepper, fresh ground

1 tbsp. fresh lemon juice

2 tbsp. balsamic vinegar, or red wine vinegar

1/2 tsp. Worcestershire sauce

3/4 tsp. kosher salt

1/8 tsp. sugar

2 tbsp. water

Directions:

1. Chop all the greens very, very fine (almost minced).
2. Arrange in rows in a chilled salad bowl.
3. Cut the tomatoes in half, seed, and chop very fine.
4. Fine dice the turkey, avocado, eggs, and bacon.
5. Arrange all the ingredients, including the blue cheese, in rows across the lettuces.
6. Sprinkle with the chives.
7. Present at the table in this fashion, then toss with the dressing at the very last minute and serve in chilled salad bowls.
8. Serve with fresh French bread.
9. **For the Dressing:** Combine all the ingredients except the olive oil in a blender and blend.
10. Slowly, with the machine running, add the oil and blend well.
11. Keep refrigerated.
12. **Note:** This dish should be kept chilled and served as chilled as possible.

5.6 Mediterranean Gnocchi

Cooking Time:	Servings:	Difficulty:
5'	2	Easy

Ingredients:

1 bag fresh gnocchi
9 oz. mixed grilled vegetables—
peppers, aubergines, courgettes
and dried tomatoes
2 tbsp. red pesto

3 or 4 basil leaves
Grated parmesan

Directions:

1. In a large pot, boil some salted water. As soon as it boils, add the gnocchi and cook for 2 minutes.
2. When the gnocchi rises to the surface, drain and put them back in the pot together with a drop of the cooking water.
3. Add the vegetables, cut into small pieces, the red pesto, and basil.
4. Serve after sprinkling with Parmesan.

5.7 Mediterranean Pasta with Basil

Cooking Time:	Servings:	Difficulty:
30'	4	Easy

Ingredients:

About 12 oz. pasta

2 lb. cherry tomatoes cut in quarters

2 red peppers cut into small pieces and without seeds

2 red chilies cut into cubes and without seeds

2 red onions cut into wedges

3 minced garlic cloves

2 tbsp. olive oil

1 tsp. sugar

5 or 6 fresh basil leaves

Grated Parmesan cheese

Directions:

1. Preheat the oven to 390°F/350°F.
2. Arrange the peppers, chilies, onions, and garlic in a large enough pan. Sprinkle with sugar and season with oil, salt, and pepper.
3. Bake for 18 minutes, then add the tomatoes and cook for another 15 minutes until lightly browned.
4. Meanwhile, cook the pasta in a large saucepan with salted water.
5. Remove the vegetables from the oven and pour the pasta into the pan, stirring slightly.
6. Serve sprinkling with the broken basil leaves and Parmesan cheese.

5.8 Rice with Tomato and Basil

Cooking Time:	Servings:	Difficulty:
25'	4	Easy

Ingredients:

1 tbsp. butter
1 tbsp. olive oil
3 finely sliced brown shallots
1 celery stalk finely diced
2 cup arborio rice
½ cup white wine
2 ½ pt. light chicken or vegetable broth

2 thinly diced courgettes
2 large ripe red tomatoes
1 tbsp. extra-virgin olive oil
sea salt and pepper
2 tbsp. of basil leaves for serving
freshly grated parmesan, to serve
1 pinch chili sauce

Directions:

1. In a large pot with a very thick bottom, melt the butter and oil and add the shallot and celery, stirring to soften.
2. Add the rice and mix slowly until everything is smooth.
3. Still stirring, now add the white wine and boil until absorbed for about 2 minutes
4. Add all but a ladle of broth and bring to a boil.
5. Turn the heat to low, cover, and cook gently for about 18 minutes.
6. Then add the remaining stock and diced courgettes. Let it go for another 5 minutes.
7. Cut the tomatoes in half, remove the seeds, and then dice everything.
8. In the end, add the tomatoes and season with olive oil, salt, and pepper. Before serving, sprinkle with basil leaves and grated Parmesan cheese.

5.9 Lemony Mushroom Pilaf

Cooking Time:	Servings:	Difficulty:
50'	8	Easy

Ingredients:

1 onion, finely chopped

1 tbsp. vegetable oil

1 tsp. garam masala

1 tsp. cumin, ground

1 tsp. tomato purée

5 oz. red lentils, washed and drained

½ in. piece ginger, finely chopped

2 garlic cloves, crushed

8 oz. bag spinach leaves, chopped

8 oz. basmati rice

Peppers

1 ½ pt. vegetable stock

Handful mint leaves, chopped

Directions:

1. In a big saucepan with a filter, heat the oil. Cook for 5 minutes until the garlic, onion, and ginger have softened. Cook for 1 minute more after adding the tomato spices and purée. Pour throughout the stock and stir to coat the rice. Bring to a boil, and then add the lentils, cover, and cook on low heat for 15 minutes, or until the lentils and rice are cooked. Mix the spinach with mint in a bowl and mix.

2. Remove the tops of each pepper with a sharp knife. Cut a middle stalk and any seeds with a knife. Trim the bottom slightly, so they remain upright, but not so far that the filling falls out. Fill every pepper with the rice mixture and cover with the lid. Bake or you can freeze it firmly wrapped in cling film or foil pouches.

3. If using frozen peppers, defrost entirely before cooking. Preheat oven to 390°F/350°F fan/gas mark 6. Place the peppers on a baking tray (gently oiled) and bake for 25-30 minutes or until softened. Toss a green salad with cucumber, herbs, and a spoonful of yogurt before serving.

5.11 Carrot and Coriander pilaf

Cooking Time:	Servings:	Difficulty:
30'	4	Easy

Ingredients:

1 tbsp. butter

1 tbsp. vegetable oil

1 small onion, finely chopped

1 tbsp. mustard seeds

1 tsp. ground coriander

1 tsp. coriander seeds

1 tsp. turmeric

1 tsp. cumin seeds

1 cup rinsed basmati rice

1 cup grated carrot

2 cup water

1 lemon, quartered

1 tsp. salt

Directions:

1. In a saucepan with a lid, heat the oil and cook the onion. Add all the spices and wait 1 minute before adding the grated carrot.
2. Add the water, rice, and salt and bring to a boil, stirring.
3. Put the heat on low, cover the saucepan tightly and simmer for about 15 minutes.
4. When ready, leave to rest covered for 5 minutes and then serve with the lemon wedges and fresh coriander.

5.12 Spiced Carrot and Lentil Soup

Cooking Time:	Servings:	Difficulty:
15'	4	Easy

Ingredients:

½ cup milk (fat-free)

5 oz. red lentils, split

2 tbsp. olive oil

2 tsp. cumin seeds

1 ¼ lbs. carrots, coarsely grated,

but no need to peel

Hot vegetable stock, cube

Pinch chili flakes

Plain yogurt and naan bread for serving

Directions:

1. Dry-fry 2 tsp. cumin seeds as well as a pinch of the chili flakes in a big saucepan for 1 minute, or before they start to hop around and unleash their aromas.
2. Using a spoon, scoop out about half of the mixture and put it aside. Bring 2 tsp. olive oil, 1 ¼ lb. thinly sliced grated carrots, 5 oz. split red lentils, 2-pints hot vegetable stock, and ½ cup milk to a boil in a saucepan.
3. Cook for 15 minutes, or until the lentils are softened and darkened.
4. Using a stick blender or a food processor, puree the soup until creamy (or, if you prefer, leave it chunky).
5. Season to taste, then top with a dollop of yogurt as well as a sprinkling of the toasted spices that were set aside. Hot naan or bread is a great accompaniment.

5.13 Broccoli and Green Kale Soup

Cooking Time:	Servings:	Difficulty:
20'	2	Easy

Ingredients:

½ tsp. coriander, ground

1 lime, zested and juiced

1 tbsp. sunflower oil

3 ½ oz. kale, chopped

2 garlic cloves, sliced

7 oz. courgette, roughly sliced

1 in. piece turmeric root, grated

1/2 tsp. turmeric, ground

1 pt. stock (formed by mixing 1

tbsp. bouillon powder and jug boiled water)

3 oz. broccoli

Pinch pink Himalayan salt

Small pack parsley, roughly chopped (but reserve the few whole leaves for serving)

Thumb-sized piece ginger, sliced

Directions:

1. In a deep skillet, heat the oil and add ginger, garlic, turmeric, coriander, and salt. Cook for 2 minutes on medium heat, and then add 3 tbsp. water to moisten the spices.
2. Stir in the courgette; make sure they are properly coated in all of the ingredients, then cook for another 3 minutes. Simmer for 3 minutes after adding ¾ pt. stock.
3. Pour the remaining stock over the kale, broccoli, and lime juice. Cook for another 3 to 4 minutes, or until all of the vegetables are tender.
4. Remove the pan from the heat and stir in the chopped parsley. Blend everything in a high-powered blender until smooth. Lime zest and parsley are optional for garnishing.

5.14 Creamy Pumpkin and Lentil Soup

Cooking Time:	Servings:	Difficulty:
35'	2	Easy

Ingredients:

Pinch salt and sugar

About 1 ¾ lbs. pumpkin flesh, chopped plus the seeds

2 oz. crème fraiche, plus extra to serve

2 onions, chopped

2 garlic cloves chopped

2 pt. hot vegetable stock

3 ½ oz. split red lentil

1 tbsp. olive oil, plus 1 tsp.

½ small pack thyme, leaves picked

Directions:

1. In a large dish, heat the oil. Fry fresh onions until they are softened and golden. Pour in the hot stock after whisking in the garlic, pumpkin flesh, lentils, and thyme. Season with salt and pepper, cover, cook for 20-25 minutes, or until the lentils and vegetables become soft.

2. In the meantime, clean the pumpkin seeds. Remove any remaining flesh, and then pat them dry with kitchen paper. In a non-stick skillet, heat 1 tsp. oil and fry the seeds until they appear to hop and pop. Stir constantly; however, cover the pan while stirrings to keep the ingredients protected. Add a touch of sugar and a sprinkling of salt when the seeds appear nutty and toasted, and mix well.

3. Whizz the pumpkin (cooked) mixture until creamy, then apply whizzing again and crème Fraiche. Season to taste.

4. Garnish with a dollop of crème Fraiche, a scattering of toasted seeds, and a few thyme leaves.

5.15 Moroccan Chickpea Soup

Cooking Time:	Servings:	Difficulty:
20'	4	Easy

Ingredients:

Zest and juice of ½ lemon

Large handful coriander, or parsley and flatbread for serving

2 cups hot vegetable stock

14.5 oz plum tomatoes with garlic, chopped

14.5 oz. chickpeas, rinsed and drained

2 tsp. cumin, ground

2 celery sticks, chopped

3 ½ oz. broad beans, frozen

1 tbsp. olive oil

1 onion, chopped

Directions:

1. In a big saucepan, heat the oil and gently fry the onion and celery for 10 minutes, or until softened, stirring constantly. Add the cumin and cook for another minute.
2. Increase the heat to high, and add the stock, tomatoes, and chickpeas, along with a generous pinch of black pepper. Cook for 8 minutes. Cook for another 2 minutes after adding the broad beans and lemon juice. Season with salt and pepper, then garnish with lemon zest and the chopped herbs. With flatbread, if desired.

5.16 Mediterranean Chunky Tomato Soup

Cooking Time:	Servings:	Difficulty:
40'	4	Easy

Ingredients:

1 vegetable stock cube, reduced-salt

2 tbsp. garlic, chopped

14.5 oz. can tomato, chopped

14.5 oz. vegetable mix, frozen and grilled (aubergine, onion, peppers, courgette)

2 oz. ricotta per person (basil, spread on a slice of rye bread and beaten with snipped chives)

Handful basil leaves

Directions:

1. In a large non-stick skillet, heat half of the vegetables and the garlic over high heat, constantly stirring, until they begin to soften, around 5 minutes. Add the basil, onions, stock cube, and 2 cans of water, and blitz the mixture with a hand blender until it's as smooth as possible.

2. Add the frozen vegetables, cover, and cook for another 15-20 minutes, or until the vegetables are tender. Pour into serving dishes. On rye bread, spread the herby ricotta and serve.

5.17 Chunky Butternut Mulligatawny

Cooking Time:	Servings:	Difficulty:
40'	6	Easy

Ingredients:

Black pepper

Small pack parsley, chopped

Natural yogurt to serve

3 celery sticks, finely chopped

2-3 heaped tbsp. gluten-free curry powder, depending on the extent of spiciness

2 × 14.5 oz. cans tomatoes, chopped

2 tbsp. olive or rapeseed oil

2 onions, finely chopped

2 dessert apples, peeled and finely chopped

5 oz. basmati rice

1 tbsp. nigella seeds (also known as a black onion or the kalonji seeds)

1 tbsp. cinnamon, ground

1 ½ lbs. gluten-free chicken or vegetable stock

½ small butternut squash, peeled, chopped into small pieces, seeds removed

Option: 3 tbsp. mango chutney, plus a little to serve

Directions:

1. In the biggest saucepan, heat the oil. With a sprinkle of flour, toss in the onions, apples, and celery. Cook and stir for 10 minutes, or until softened. Mix the butternut squash, cinnamon, nigella seeds, curry powder, and black pepper pinch in a mixing bowl. Cook for another 2 minutes, then add the tomatoes and stock. Simmer for 15 minutes with the cover on.

2. The vegetables must be soft but not mushy at this stage. Stir in the rice, cover, and continue to cook for another 12 minutes or until the rice is tender. If necessary, season with more salt and pepper. Stir in the parsley and mango chutney, and then serve in bowls with extra mango chutney and yogurt on top, if desired."

5.18 Acquacotta

Cooking Time:	Servings:	Difficulty:
40'	4	Easy

Ingredients:

1 red onion, finely chopped

2 garlic cloves, finely chopped

2 small carrots, chopped

2 tbsp. parsley, chopped

2 tsp. thyme leaves, plus extra to serve

8 oz. plum tomatoes, deseeded and chopped

3 celery sticks, chopped

3 slices crusty bread, toasted and torn into chunks

3 tbsp. olive oil

2 oz. porcini mushrooms, dried

6 eggs

1 ½ pt. chicken stock

Directions:

1. In a big saucepan, heat the olive oil and gently cook the celery, onion, garlic, carrots, and thyme for bout 10-15 minutes, or until it becomes softened. Meanwhile, soak the porcini for 15 minutes in hot water until softened and swollen. Drain the mushrooms and finely cut them, reserving the soaking juice. Cook for another 5 minutes with the softened vegetables and the soaking liquid.
2. Add the tomatoes, then cook for 10 minutes, or before they start to break down, and add the stock, then bring to a slow boil.
3. In another large saucepan, poach the 6 eggs for 3-4 minutes, or until set, now remove with the slotted spoon. Toss in the parsley and a pinch of salt and pepper, as well as torn up the toasted bread. Distribute the soup among 6 bowls and top each with an egg. Serve with a sprinkling of fresh thyme.

5.19 Griddled Vegetable and Feta Tart

Cooking Time:	Servings:	Difficulty:
40'	4	Easy

Ingredients:

1 aubergine, sliced

1 tsp. oregano, dried

10-12 cherry tomatoes, halved

2 courgette, sliced

2 red onions, chunky wedges

2 tbsp. olive oil

3 large sheets filo pastry

3 oz. feta cheese, crumbled

A drizzle balsamic vinegar

Low-fat dressing and a large bag of mixed salad leaves, to serve

Directions:

1. Preheat the oven to 350°F and place a 13x9-inch baking tray inside. Griddle the aubergines when nicely charred in a griddle pan with around 1 tsp. oil, then peel. Using a little more oil if necessary, repeat with both the courgette and onions.

2. Take the tray out of the oven and lightly oil it. Brush a big sheet of filo with oil, layer another sheet on top, drizzle with some more oil, and repeat with a final sheet. Place the pastry on the hot tray and gently press it into the corners.

3. Arrange the griddled vegetables on top, then season with salt and pepper. Drizzle the vinegar and any leftover oil over the tomatoes, cut-side up. Sprinkle oregano and crumbled feta on top. Cook for about 20 minutes, or until golden and crispy. Serve with the blended salad leaves that have been dressed.

5.20 Spinach, Mushroom and Potato Pie

Cooking Time:	Servings:	Difficulty:
45'	4	Easy

Ingredients:

1 tbsp. grain mustard

1 tbsp. olive oil

1 tsp. freshly nutmeg, grated

2 garlic cloves, crushed

2 heaped tbsp. light crème Fraiche

1 cup vegetable stock

3 sheets filo pastry

10 oz. new potatoes, cooked and cut as bite-sized pieces

10 oz, green beans and broccoli, steamed

14.5 oz. baby spinach

1 lb. mushroom, like shiitake, chestnut, and button

Directions:

1. Preheat the oven to 390°F/350°F fan/gas 6. In a colander, wilt spinach by pouring a bowl of warm water over it.
2. In a big nonstick skillet, heat half of the oil and cook the mushrooms until golden brown. Cook for 1 minute after adding the garlic, and then add the stock, mustard, nutmeg, and potatoes. Boil for few minutes or before the volume is decreased. Season with salt and pepper, then extract from the heat; stir in the spinach and crème Fraiche. Enable to cool in a pie dish for a few minutes.
3. Brush the remaining oil on the filo sheets, quarter them, then scrunch them up and position them on top of the pie filling. Bake for 20-25 minutes, or until golden brown. Serve along with vegetables.

5.21 Paillard Chicken with Lemon and Herbs

Cooking Time:	Servings:	Difficulty:
20'	6	Easy

Ingredients:

½ tbsp. balsamic vinegar

5 oz. bag rocket

2 tbsp. olive oil

1 oz. parmesan

Chicken breasts, skinless

Lemon wedges

For the marinade:

2 garlic cloves

3 rosemary sprigs, finely chopped leaves

Sage leaves, finely shredded

1 lemon juice and zest

3 tbsp. olive oil

Directions:

1. Every chicken breast should be sandwiched between 2 sheets of cling film or baking parchment. Flatten each chicken piece with a meat mallet or rolling pin to an even layer about 1/5 in. thick. Place in a serving bowl.
2. To create the marinade, use a pestle and mortar to grind the garlic with a pinch of salt. Add the rosemary and sage and pound altogether. Combine the lemon juice, olive oil, and freshly ground black pepper in a mixing cup. Pour the marinade over the chicken to make sure it's fully covered. Refrigerate for at least 2 hours after coating.
3. Preheat the barbecue. Add coals. Cook for 1-2 minutes on either side of the chicken. Shift to a board and set aside for a few minutes to cool.
4. In a big mixing cup, combine the oil and balsamic vinegar. Season with salt and pepper and add the rocket. Mix all together, then shave the Parmesan on top. Serve the salad with chicken and lemon wedges for squeezing.

1. 22 Spanish chicken with garlic and fresh bay leaves

Cooking Time:	Servings:	Difficulty:
40'	4	Easy

Ingredients:

2 whole breasts and 2 whole chicken legs

4 tbsp. olive oil

6 fresh bay leaves

2 garlic bulbs

1 glass Sherry

Directions:

1. Cut the chicken breasts in half. Season the chicken with salt.
2. In a large, deep saucepan with a thick bottom and an airtight lid, heat the oil. Fry the garlic cloves over medium heat and when they turn slightly golden, remove and set aside. Fry the chicken until golden brown on all sides, about 5 minutes for each piece. Eliminate excess fat.
3. Put the garlic back into the pot together with the bay leaf and pour the Sherry.
4. Add a little oil and simmer for about two minutes, turning the chicken continuously in its sauce.
5. Now add ½ cup of water, close the pot with the lid and simmer for 4 minutes. The thighs will take longer to cook, so as soon as the chicken breasts are ready, remove them and set them aside.
6. Continue to cook the remaining chicken as long as needed, adding water to the sauce if necessary. Then reinsert the chicken breasts to warm them up.
7. Serve with pilaf and seasonal vegetables. Finish your party with Neil Perry's Spanish Quince Almond Pie.

5.23 Teriyaki Salmon Parcels

Cooking Time:	Servings:	Difficulty:
20'	4	Easy

Ingredients:

2 tbsp. low-salt soy sauce

1 tbsp. clear honey

1 garlic clove, finely chopped

A little sunflower oil

10 oz. Tenderstem broccoli

4×3 ½ oz. salmon fillets

1 small ginger piece, cut into matchsticks

1 tbsp butter

Spring onions, sliced (toasted sesame seeds)

Rice, cooked for serving

Optional:

A little sesame oil

1 tbsp. mirin

Directions:

1. Prepare the marinade and sauce. Set aside a little bowl containing the soy sauce, butter, garlic, and mirin.
2. Cut some foil squares out. Cut 4 squares of aluminum foil, each about 12 in. square, with scissors. Brush a little oil onto each sheet of foil to pull the edges up a little.
3. Fill the parcels to the maximum. Place a few broccoli stems on top of each one, then a salmon fillet and ginger on top.
4. Pour the sauce on top. Pour the sauce on each salmon fillet and, if desired, drizzle with
5. sesame oil.
6. Close the packs. To seal the parcels, fold the foil edges together and position them on a baking sheet. It's possible to schedule it up to a day ahead of time.
7. Prepare the parcels. Preheat oven to 390°F.
8. Let cook the parcels for 15-20 minutes, then removes them and leaves them to cool for a few minutes. Place each packet on the plate and open it. Serve with rice on the side and a sprinkle of spring onions and sesame seeds."

5.24 Sea Bass with Chili Sizzled Ginger and Spring Onions

Cooking Time:	Servings:	Difficulty:
30'	6	Easy

Ingredients:

6 sea bass fillets (5 oz. each with skin and scaled)

3 tbsp. sunflower oil

Large ginger knob, peeled and shredded in matchsticks

3 garlic cloves, thinly sliced

3 fresh red chilies, deseeded and thinly shredded

Bunch spring onion, shredded long-ways

1 tbsp. soy sauce

Directions:

1. Salt and pepper 6 sea bass fillets, then slash a skin 3 times.
2. Heat 1 tbsp. sunflower oil in a heavy-bottomed frying pan.
3. When the oil is heated, fry the sea bass fillets while keeping the skin-side down for 5 minutes, or when the skin is crisp and golden. The fish will be almost completely fried.
4. Flip and cook for a further 30 seconds to 1 minute before transferring to a serving plate to stay warm. The sea bass fillets can be fried in 2 batches.
5. In a big skillet, heat 2 tsp. sunflower oil, and fry the big knob of peeled ginger, 3 garlic cloves (thinly sliced), and 3 red chilies (thinly shredded) for about 2 mins or until golden, then cut into matchsticks,
6. Remove the pan from the heat and add the shredded spring onions.
7. Put 1 tbsp. soy sauce on the fish and spoon on the pan's contents.

5.25 Moroccan Tuna

Cooking Time:	Servings:	Difficulty:
10'	4	Easy

Ingredients:

3 crushed garlic cloves

½ tsp. paprika

½ ground cumin

½ chili powder

some coriander leaves and stalks

1 lemon juice

About half a glass olive oil

4 7 oz. fresh tuna steaks, about 1 inch. thick

Directions:

1. Put all the spices along with the garlic and lemon in a blender and reduce to a puree. Slowly add the olive oil until you have a slightly thick sauce. Let it rest.
2. Place the tuna in a ceramic dish and sprinkle it with the sauce. Cover with plastic wrap and marinate in the fridge for up to 4 hours.
3. Remove excess marinade, season the tuna, and cook for 3 minutes per side on a hot grill.
4. Sprinkle the tuna with the remaining sauce before serving.

5.26 Mama's Supper Club Tilapia Parmesan

Cooking Time:	Servings:	Difficulty:
35'	4	Easy

Ingredients:

1 dash hot pepper sauce

1/4 tsp. basil, dried

1/4 tsp. seasoning salt

3 tbsp. green onions, finely chopped

3 tbsp. mayonnaise

4 tbsp. butter, room temperature

1/2 cup parmesan cheese, grated

2 tbsp. lemon juice

2 lbs. tilapia fillets (orange cod, roughly or red snapper can be replaced)

Directions:

1. Preheat oven to 350°F.
2. Arrange the fillets in a single layer in a buttered 13 x 9-inch baking tray or jellyroll tray.
3. Fillets should not be stacked.
4. Brush the top with juice.
5. In a bowl, combine butter, mayonnaise, cheese, onions, and seasonings.
6. Mix with a fork.
7. Bake the fish for 10 to 20 minutes, or before it begins to flake.
8. Spread the cheese mixture on top and bake for 5 minutes or until golden brown.
9. The time it would take to roast the fish can be calculated by its thickness.
10. Keep an eye on the fish to make sure it doesn't overcook.
11. Note: This fish can be cooked in a broiler as well.
12. Broil for at least 3 to 4 minutes.
13. Broil for another 2 or 3 minutes, just until cheese is browned.

5.27 Ricotta, Tomato and Spinach Frittata

Cooking Time:	Servings:	Difficulty:
35'	4	Easy

Ingredients:

1 tbsp. olive oil
1 large onion, sliced
10 oz. cherry tomatoes
3 ½ oz. spinach leaves
A small handful basil leaves

3 ½ oz. ricotta
6 eggs, beaten
Salad for serving

Directions:

1. Preheat oven to 390°F or 350°F.
2. In a big non-stick frying pan, heat the oil and fry the onion for about 5-6 minutes, or until tender and golden. To soften the tomatoes, put them in for 1 minute.
3. Turn off the heat and put the spinach leaves, then basil to wilt a bit. In an oiled 13 × 9-inch rectangular baking tin, mix all of the ingredients. Dot the ricotta over the vegetables in little scoops.
4. Season the eggs and whisk them thoroughly before pouring them over the vegetables and cheese. Cook for 20 to 25 minutes in the oven or until lightly golden. Serve with a salad.

5.28 Spinach and Pepper Frittata

Cooking Time:	Servings:	Difficulty:
40'	4	Easy

Ingredients:

5 large eggs

10 oz. low-fat cottage cheese

8 oz. leaf spinach, frozen, squeezed, thawed, and finely chopped

2 red peppers, roasted, torn into strips

½ oz. parmesan or any vegetarian alternative, finely grated

3 ½ oz. whole cherry tomato

1 garlic clove, finely chopped

Grating nutmeg, generous

Directions:

1. Preheat the oven to 375°F/335°F fan/gas mark 15. If your sandwich tin has a loose rim, line it with a single sheet of baking parchment.
2. In a big mixing cup, whisk together the eggs, garlic, cottage cheese, half of the Parmesan, spinach, nutmeg, pepper, and black pepper. Fill the tray halfway with the mixture, then top with tomatoes and the leftover Parmesan. Bake about 40 minutes, or until fully set and beginning to puff up.
3. You can serve hot or cold after cutting into wedges. In the fridge, it will last 3-4 days.

5.29 Healthy Egg and Chips

Cooking Time:	Servings:	Difficulty:
1 h	4	Easy

Ingredients:

1 tbsp. olive oil

2 shallots, sliced

2 tsp. oregano, dried, crushed, or fresh leaves

7 oz. small mushroom

4 eggs

1 lb. potatoes, diced

Directions:

1. Preheat oven to 390°F/350°F fan/gas mark 6. Place the potatoes and shallots in a big non-stick roasting pan, drizzle with oil, and season with oregano, and then toss well. Bake for 40-45 minutes (or when the potatoes are beginning to brown), then add the mushrooms and cook for another 10 minutes, or until the potatoes become browned and soft.
2. Cut four holes in the vegetables, and then put the eggs into each. Return the eggs to the oven for another 3-4 minutes, or until they are fried to your taste.

5.30 Blueberry Compote with Porridge

Cooking Time:	Servings:	Difficulty:
5'	2	Easy

Ingredients:

0% fat yogurt
½ pack blueberries, frozen
A tbsp. porridge oats
Water
Optional: 1 tsp. honey

Directions:

1. In a non-stick pan, mix the oats in 1 pt. water and cook, stirring regularly, for around 2 minutes, or until thickened. Take the pan off the heat and whisk in a quarter of the yogurt.
2. In the meantime, gently poach the blueberries in a pan with 2 tsp. water and the sugar, if used, until they have thawed and are soft but still retain their form.
3. Divide the Porridge among cups, cover with the remaining yogurt, and scatter the blueberries on top.

5.31 Beetroot Mustard and Lentil Salad

Cooking Time:	Servings:	Difficulty:
20'	6	Easy

Ingredients:

1 large handful tarragon, coarsely chopped

1 packet (10 oz.) (not pickled) beetroot, sliced and cooked

1 ½ tbsp.. extra-virgin olive oil

1 tbsp. whole-grain mustard or alternatively gluten-free

7 oz. puy lentils or 2 packs of 9 oz. precooked lentils

Directions:

1. If you're not using pre-cooked lentils, cook them according to package directions, then drain and cool in a mixing bowl.
2. Meanwhile, make a dressing with mustard, oil, and tarragon.
3. Pour the dressing over the lentils and mix well.
4. Serve with the beets, tarragon, and a pinch of salt and pepper.

5.32 Potato and Paprika Tortilla

Cooking Time:	Servings:	Difficulty:
25'	4	Easy

Ingredients:

6 large eggs

3 tbsp. olive oil

9 oz. new potato, thickly sliced, ends trimmed

2 garlic cloves, chopped

1 small onion, halved and sliced

½ tsp. paprika, smoked

½ tsp. oregano, dried, or 3 tbsp. parsley, chopped

Few extra leaves for garnishing (optional)

Directions:

1. In a deep 9 inches non-stick frying pan, heat the oil. Cook the potatoes, onion, and garlic in a skillet for 10 minutes or until tender. Stir in paprika and cook for another minute.
2. Season the eggs with the dried or some fresh herbs, and then pour them into the pan. When the egg begins to set on the pan's bottom, stir about a couple of times, then cover and cook gently over a very low flame for 10 minutes, or until set, other than the top.
3. Place the tortilla on a plate with care. Transfer to the pan and an uncooked top on the surface, and cook for another 1-2 minutes. Cover in foil.
4. Serve warm or cool while garnished with parsley if desired.

5.33 Soy Sauce Spinach

Cooking Time:	Servings:	Difficulty:
10'	4	Easy

Ingredients:

1 garlic clove
1 bag spinach
2 tbsp. soy sauce
1 tbsp. vegetable oil
1 tbsp. toasted sesame seeds

Directions:

1. In a non-stick pan, heat the oil and brown the garlic for a few seconds.
2. Add the spinach and cook for 2 minutes, stirring constantly.
3. Pour the soy, mix and sprinkle with the sesame seeds. Excellent as an accompaniment to chicken or grilled.

5.34 Ramon with Sesame

Cooking Time:	Servings:	Difficulty:
15'	1	Easy

Ingredients:

1 pack instant noodles with sesame

1 egg

2 finely chopped spring onions

½ pak choi

1 teaspoon sesame seeds

chili sauce

Directions:

1. Cook the spaghetti with its herbs and when 1 minute is left to cook, add the spring onions and pak choi.
2. Boil the egg for about 6 minutes from boiling and stop cooking by passing it under cold water, then peel it.
3. Toast the sesame seeds in a pan.
4. Pour the spaghetti with spring onions and pak choi into a deep bowl, cut the hard-boiled egg in half, and place it on top of the noodles.
5. Sprinkle the whole with the sesame seeds and drizzle with the chili sauce.

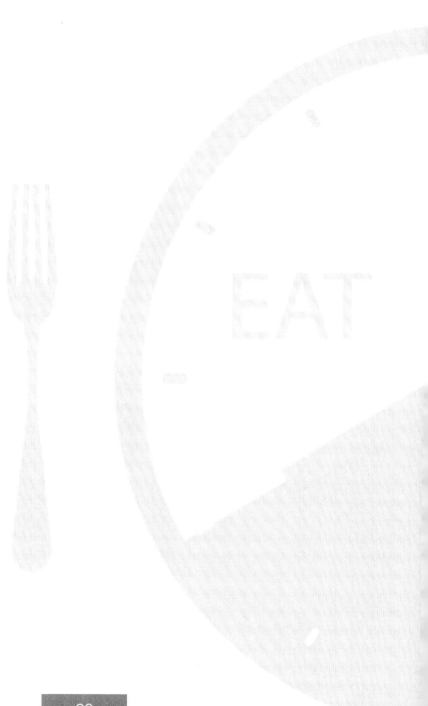

Don't Forget my Gift!!!

Once again thanks for buying my book!. If you've read the book up to this point, I'm sure you appreciated the advice I wanted to share with you, so I'd be grateful if you'd like to share your appreciation too.

Leave a 5 star review:

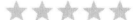

I ask you for an honest and truthful review.

This way you can help other women choose this book and embark on Intermittent Fasting.

Many thanks!

Click on the link below to get immediate access to

"The Intermittent Fasting. Weekly Plan":

https://bit.ly/fastingweeklyplan

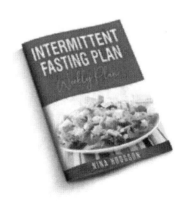

Bibliography

- Intermittent fasting for beginners, 2021, www.dietdoctor.com

- Intermittent fasting: surprising update, 2018, www.health.harvard.edu

- What's intermittent fasting? The science behind it, 2020, www.zmescience.com

- Anti-aging Benefits of Intermittent Fasting, 2016, neurohacker.com

- Study: Intermittent Fasting Works to Lose Weight AND Slow the Aging Process, 2020, thebeet.com

- The Beginner's Guide to Intermittent Fasting, jamesclear.com

- Intermittent Fasting: What is it, and how does it work?, www.hopkinsmedicine.org

- What You Need To Know About Intermittent Fasting, 2021, betterme.world

- 6 Popular Ways to Do Intermittent Fasting, www.healthline.com

- 20 Best Foods to Eat While Intermittent Fasting, 2020,

- Intermittent Fasting Meal Plan: Here's Exactly When & What To Eat, 2020, www.mindbodygreen.com

- A Complete Guide To Intermittent Fasting + Daily Plan & Schedule, 2020, 21dayhero.com

- Pros and Cons of Intermittent Fasting, 2020, www.verywellfit.com

- 7 common Intermittent Fasting Myths, debunked, www.humnutrition.com

- Intermittent Fasting? Here's How To Exercise Safely & Effectively, 2020, www.mindbodygreen.com

- 6 Things to Know About Intermittent Fasting and Working Out, www.atkins.com

- 9 Intermittent Fasting Mistakes Beginners Make (And How To Avoid Them!), www.asweetpeachef.com

- You're Probably Doing Intermittent Fasting the Wrong Way— Here's Why, 2019, www.cookinglight.com

- www.bbcgoodfood.com

Page Intentionally left blank

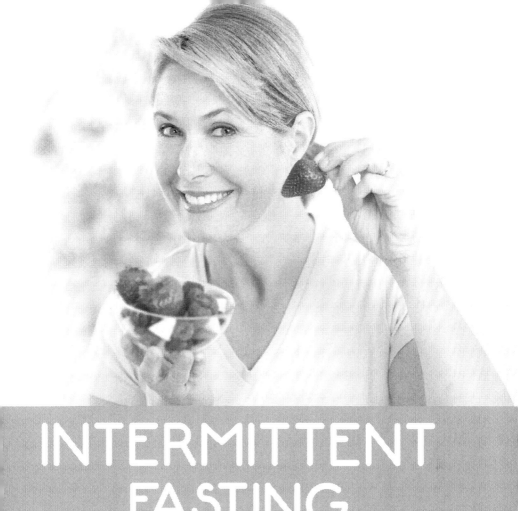

INTERMITTENT FASTING for Women over 50

14 Days to Adopt a New Healthy Lifestyle and Change Your Habits. How to Get Immediate Results, Working on Motivation to Increase Your Well-Being

Nina Hodgson

Table of Contents

Your Free Gift

Thanks for buying my book! I have prepared an exclusive gift for the readers of:

"Intermittent Fasting for Women over 50: 14 Days to Adopt a New Healthy Lifestyle and Change Your Habits. How to Get Immediate Results, Working on Motivation to Increase Your Well-Being"

Click on the link below to get immediate access to "The Intermittent Fasting Weekly Plan":

https://bit.ly/fastingweeklyplan

Once you finish reading the book, it would be great if you could leave a review on Amazon.

You know, this is very easy to do, go to the ORDERS section of your Amazon account and click on the "Write a review for the product" button. It will automatically take you to the review section.

Leave a 5 star review:

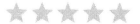

Thanks and good Intermittent Fasting!

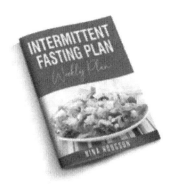

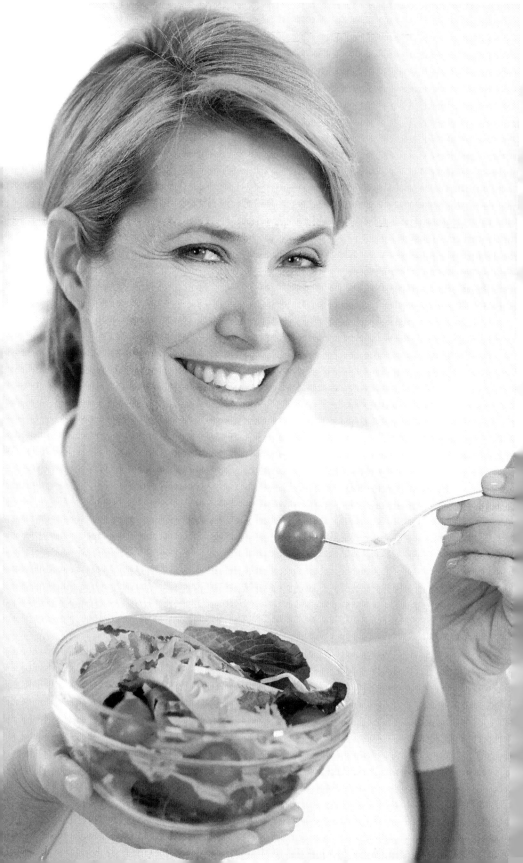

Introduction

Nina Hodgson was born in Livingston, Montana, into a family where both parents worked in the health and nutrition field. As a child, she loved running around by the lake and hiking with her family. She dreamed of being a dancer when she grew up; since that did not work for her, she decided to go into her second love, helping others feel better.

From a young age, she found nutrition interesting. The author would frequently sit for hours talking with her parents about their work, and the three of them would share ideas. As she matured, she would read books and magazines about the topic. As she got older, she saw how our culture put such emphasis on looking a specific way. Frequently, people would achieve this perfect look in ways that were unsafe and difficult to maintain.

In high school, she worked in the local library, putting away books, and arranging the card catalog (they were not always on the computer), but her favorite was when she helped her mom and dad with their work. It was no surprise when she went to college and earned a degree in Masters Nutritional Education.

For most of her life, Nina struggled with her weight. She followed the food pyramid guidelines, making sure she ate the recommended serving sizes and worked out 30 minutes a day. While this seemed logical, it did not always leave her feeling, her best, and her weight would still fluctuate. She would see the same types of frustrations with her clients and was not sure how to help.

In the early 90s, many different diet plans promised to increase energy and help you lose weight and feel better. These diet plans paired with Jane Fonda workouts seemed the perfect way to stay on track. Some diets were so restrictive that you could only eat one food, such as the cottage cheese diet and cabbage soup diet. Other diets were unhealthy due to the food restrictions, such as the Beverly Hills diet, where you could only eat fruits. There was also the liquid diet that was extremely unhealthy. Once you went back to eating normally on each of these diets, you would gain the weight right back.

Nothing seemed to work, and Nina was becoming more and more discouraged and developed a love/hate relationship with food. A large part of this love-hate relationship comes from attempting to follow the guidelines and them not working correctly for everyone. People like Nina believed what textbooks and the leading researchers said about how to live a healthy lifestyle.

She was tired of trying to deal with what the researchers recommended as a nutritional diet. She started reading every book and article she could find about different body types and that eating was not a one size fits all kind of thing, but instead, it had to work for your body type or be inclusive for multiple body types.

She toured around the United States doing many seminars regarding how diet and nutrition were not one size fits all or a quick fix; you have to find a healthy way of life that you enjoy and that works with your daily life.

As she entered her 40s and 50s, she found that there wasn't much information about nutrition for these ages. Nina knew that the same nutrition guidelines would not work for women in their 50s as they did for women in their 20s and 30s. Helping women fifty and older became her new goal.

Nina tried many different recommended diets and had a difficult time being able to maintain them. Some of them did not include enough food varieties or cut out the meals she enjoyed. They would recommend workouts that didn't target the areas she wanted to achieve or ones that left her in a lot of pain the next day. It was not the diets themselves that were not good, but instead, they were not the right fit for her.

Women over 50, like all people, must find a diet that they can maintain long term. It may not look the same as your friends or a family member. The diet should include foods you enjoy that make you feel good and provide for your nutritional needs. When choosing a diet, look for one that suits your personal needs. Are you trying to lose weight? Do you want to feel better? Do you want a healthier lifestyle, or do you simply want to maintain your energy levels as you age?

Nina discovered that there are specific dietary needs for women over 50. These women have to ensure that they are getting enough calcium for bone health. Vitamin D helps absorb calcium and maintain muscle health. Protein gives you energy and also helps with the vitamins B absorption which is essential for overall good health and helps with energy.

Nina's first book, "Intermittent Fasting for Women over 50: A Guide to Intermittent Fasting and Increasing Your Metabolism and Energy Levels. The Best Healthy Way to Detox Your Body and Rejuvenate" resulted from many years of struggling to find healthy options for women her age. She was excited to write both of these books for women, like herself, frustrated with trying to find a healthy way of life. In her first book, she touched on how intermittent fasting works in detail. The short answer to this is a daily diet where you fast for a specific amount of time and eat in a particular amount of time. During the eating time, you do not gorge yourself but instead, focus on eating healthy. Some people forget that you should enjoy your food; it is not just about what you put into your body but how you feel about what you put into your body.

Intermittent fasting can help to reduce your chances of various health problems. Obesity is the cause of many health problems. By losing weight and regulating insulin, it may lower your chance of having heart-related disorders and diabetes. It is important to note that, like any new diet, it is essential to talk to your doctor first.

After writing her first book, Nina was excited to start her second one using more of what she learned to further help women. This book will give you a quick recap about IF, what it is, and its advantages. The second half of the book focuses more on healthier lifestyles that are achievable.

This book gives you 2 detailed 14-day diet plans to help you jump-start your new way of living. You will get to see precisely what the author did to kick start her journey with IF. In this book, you will be told the daily exercises Nina did to reach her best self. If you are looking for some great recipes to go along with your new lifestyle, you should get Nina's first book. The book contains an entire chapter full of 34 delicious food ideas.

If you haven't done so yet, click here and buy the book.

Nina did the 14-day eating plan and felt great. She is now in her 3rd year of living this way and has never felt better. She uses the 16:8 fasting plan. This is simply fasting for 16 hours and eating for 8. While this sounds difficult, the majority of the time, you are sleeping. She now feels good about herself, her weight is no longer fluctuating, and she has energy.

Nina is married with 2 adult children and 1 grandchild. She believes there is nothing better than being a grandmother. She still lives in Livingston, Montana, and owns 2 acres, which they use to grow fresh fruit. She learned from all her research the importance of fresh, whole foods instead of processed foods that are high in chemicals.

There are plenty of books on this subject on the market, thanks again for choosing this one! Every effort was made to ensure it is full of as much useful information as possible. Please enjoy!

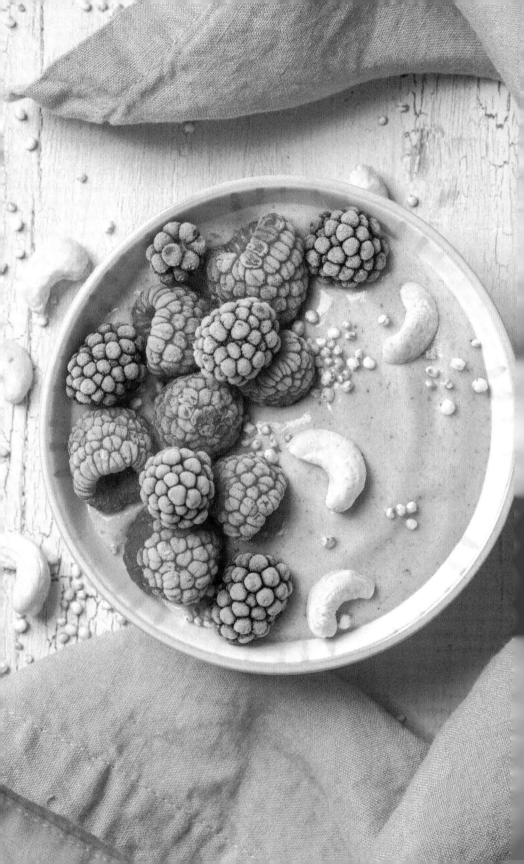

1

Fundamentals of Intermittent Fasting

1.1 WHAT IS INTERMITTENT FASTING?

We have all heard of fasting; people have been doing it since the beginning of time. Some have fasted for religious purposes, tests of strength, or other types of ceremonies. While the concept is similar between the two, there is one main difference. The intermittent fasting we are going to talk about is considered a way to turn unhealthy eating habits into healthier ones.

Currently, this is one of the most popular healthy eating plans that people are starting to use. While there have not been many studies on IF, some, like the one from Healthline, show that it does help women lose weight. Weight loss occurs because you eat fewer calories and burn more due to the eating and fasting cycle.

Intermittent fasting (IF) is when you alternate hours between eating and fasting. It is not considered a diet but instead is an eating plan. The difference between the two is that one is a short-term diet focused on weight loss. An eating plan or meal plan is not focused entirely on losing weight but on a long-term change.

There are many different ways you can do intermittent fasting. Some do it daily for a specific number of hours, others do it every other day, and others twice a week. This all sounds pretty simple, right? Those days of fasting are difficult at first. It takes real willpower not to eat. During challenging times, I would get a glass of water, put lemon and lime in it, then drink it slowly.

With IF, there are no specialty diets you have to follow. You do not have to count carbs or calories, making this an easy-to-follow lifestyle change. While there is no list of foods you should or should not eat, it is best not to binge eat on your non-fasting days. If you do binge on the non-fasting day, you will not feel great the following day. While on your fast, you should not eat, but you want to keep your calories 400 or less if you have to.

Celebrities are also using IF as a healthy way of eating. Even if they do not need to lose weight, they like how it makes them feel. After eating this way for a few weeks, many people start noticing a difference in how they look and feel.

They begin to feel like they have more energy, can think more clearly, and can get a restful night's sleep. I have also noticed that while I have not lost much weight, I am leaner.

For women over 50, intermittent fasting can be very beneficial. As we age, our bodies go through changes, especially during pre-and post-menopause. Our hormones and bodies are changing at a rapid pace causing a change in mental health. Some of these changes may cause hot flashes, mood swings, difficulty sleeping, weight gain, and depression. A study published in the Journal of Midlife Health has shown that it may offer some relief while IF will not cure them.

Weight loss is an advantage of IF. Many people are spending time eating mindlessly while sitting in front of a television or playing video games; this makes it difficult, if not impossible, to stay at a healthy weight. Christie Williams, M.S., R.D.N from John Hopiks states that portions are larger than previous years, causing more difficulty keeping a healthy weight.

Obesity is the leading cause of heart disease, stroke, high blood pressure, and can cause diabetes. IF can help to lower your risks due to not taking in as many calories and having a resting period between meals.

A few studies have shown that IF has a positive effect on cognitive function and improving memory. According to the National Library of Medicine, fasting has been shown to reduce oxidative stress. Oxidative stress is what occurs when oxygen production in the body causes tissue damage. According to BioMed Research International, a study conducted on mature weight lifters showed that IF not only improved memory but also decreased moodiness and improved mental flexibility. There were brain scans before and after the trial showing that there were actual brain structure changes.

 Most of us have experienced that midday brain fog. With intermittent fasting, people have stated that they do not experience that as frequently.

According to the Diet Doctor, this is due to a brain recycling process called autophagy. This process is fascinating; when cells become old and no longer working well, the body basically eats them. Once they are ingested, the body then produces new healthy cells to take their place.

Fasting has also been shown to benefit your skin. A study from Curr Gastroenterol Rep in 2010 states when you give your digestive system a break, it starts to renew intestinal stem cells.

Intestinal stem cells are a large part of the digestive system; without them, your body will not digest food, and it should—the probiotics found in yogurt help keep your gut healthy, which helps with skin hydration.

Inflammation is the leading cause of many health issues. IF also helps to alleviate symptoms of some chronic disorders you already have. Reducing the number of calories that are consumed helps reduce inflammation. Mount Sinai researchers stated there are cells called monocytes that increase inflammation in the body. When individuals are fasting, these cells stop circulating through the bloodstream reducing inflation. Along with the oxidative stress that I wrote about earlier, monocyte cells also cause tissue damage.

Lowering the inflammation in the body can help prevent Alzheimer's Disease. There is no cure for this disease, so prevention is the key. The Alzheimer's Prevention Institute studied animals that show a reduction in brain inflammation. Reducing inflammation helps to decrease the chances of Parkinson's and Alzheimer's disease. There has not been human research in this area, but there have been excellent results in mice. Nevertheless, IF has shown that reducing inflammation also benefits preexisting conditions such as rheumatoid arthritis, diabetes, blood pressure, etc.

The National Library of Medicine showed that IF might decrease cancer risk, help improve chemotherapy results and reduce side effects for those receiving chemo. While there have been limited human trials, the ones on mice have had promising results.

While intermittent fasting is a simple way to eat, you can be making mistakes without even realizing it. When you notice you are not getting the results you want, or perhaps when a friend and you are fasting together without getting the results you want, maybe you have to look at what you are doing.

One mistake many people make is jumping from eating every 2-4 hours right into a 24 hour fast. Not only are you going to be miserable during this time, but your body is also going not to react well. It is essential to listen to your body no matter what type of lifestyle change you will make. Start gradually, maybe try to fast for 10-12 hours, and increase the amount of fasting time you can. Another mistake that some people make is eating the wrong foods or too much food during their feasting time—one of the goals many people have when starting IF is to lose weight and become healthier.

We may overeat during our feasting window as a way of congratulating ourselves for making it through the fasting time. We may not realize the number of calories we are consuming when we are eating.

In addition to the number of calories, you may want to consider the time of the day you are eating. If you eat all of your food at night, it may trigger binge eating. In addition to binge eating too many calories at night can cause difficulty sleeping and disturb your circadian rhythms.

The opposite of eating too many calories can also be a mistake. If you do not eat enough calories, your body will start to lose muscle mass. It also throws off your metabolism, and it will start slowing down, impeding your weight-loss goals and other health-related goals.

Carbs, who doesn't love them? One mistake is when people overindulge in carbs when they eat. Carbs are tricky. You can look at the number of carbs in something and overlook their calories or understand serving sizes. I did this with oreo cookies. I know who thinks cookies are a healthy way of eating; me, that's who. If you look at the back of the package, it says serving size three cookies, 160 calories, and 25 grams of carbs. Sounds great until you look at the sodium content and the ingredients. This is just an example of a mistake I made at the start of IF.

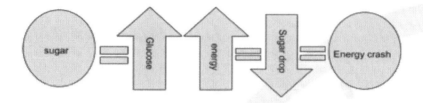

Another common mistake people make is not getting enough fluids; not drinking enough fluids while fasting can cause cramps and headaches that continue for a few days.

When fasting, you are not getting hydration from the food you usually eat, so it is easy to miss. Another thing to consider often, our feelings of hunger come from thirst. Perhaps drinking when you feel hungry may ease that feeling.

1.4 DIFFERENT INTERMITTENT FASTING TYPES AND BENEFITS

There are many types of IF. Each one contains a different number of hours to fast and hours to feast. While each is different, they have the same goal, to help you feel better and positively change your lifestyle. Below you will find a short introduction to a few different types; if you would like more information, read "**Intermittent Fasting for Women over 50: A Guide to Intermittent Fasting and Increasing Your Metabolism and Energy Levels. The Best Healthy Way to Detox Your Body and Rejuvenate**".

14:10

This plan is when you fast for 14 hours then eat for 10. This is one of the best fasting plans for women. You can eat from 10 A.M. until 8 P.M. and then fast from 8 P.M. to 10 A.M. If you love to eat breakfast, this plan may not be for you.

16:8

This is a plan where you fast for 16 hours then feast for 8 hours. This is the one that seems to have the best results for men. You simply eat from 11 A.M. to 7 P.M. This one is a great plan to start with.

20:4

In this plan, you fast for 20 hours and eat for 4 hours. To start, you can fast from 6:00 P.M. and then eat from 2:00 P.M. to 6:00 P.M.

Alternate day fasting

When I first started fasting, I thought this was the only one available. This diet is where you go 24-36 hours without eating and then eat one meal a day. With this eating plan, it is difficult to get enough calories or nutrients with one meal.

Weekly intermittent fasting

Much like it sounds, you are fasting 2-3 times a week. With this type of fasting, you are less likely to lose weight. Even though you are not expected to lose weight, you will still get health benefits.

Eat-stop-eat

This plan is fast for 2 days and eats normally for the other 5. On fasting days, you consume less than 400 calories a day for a woman and 500 calories a day for a man. Then on the days, you are not fasting, you eat normally.

Spontaneous meal skipping

This is an eating plan where you just eat when you feel hungry. There is no reason you have to eat every few hours, so when you are not hungry or do not feel like eating, just skip a meal. The only thing to remember is when you skip a meal, make sure and get the added nutrition with your next one.

The warrior diet

Is where you have 20 hours of fasting 4 hours of feasting. Ori Hofmekler created the warrior diet in the early 2000s. He started this eating plan using what he found worked best for him. The foods should be whole fresh foods and focus on eating proteins and fats. This is not a hard-fast rule but what Ori suggests. During the fasting time, you should eat very few calories, and during the feasting time, you should consume 80% of your calorie intake. This diet is not for everyone.

2

Intermittent Fasting Tricks and Tips

2.1 START SLOWLY

The first tip you should know is not to jump right into fasting but instead start slow. Many people like to decide to start something new and then just start it. If you start this way, it will be harder for you. If you ease slowly into the Fasting, your body will be able to adapt easier, and you will not be as stressed.

2.2 DO NOT COMPLICATE YOUR EATING PLAN

Do not overcomplicate this eating plan. IF is simply you eat for a bit, then you do not eat for a bit. The entire IF approach is based on the 2 things above, and you get to choose when.

Do not worry if you eat an hour before your fasting ends or eat an hour later. 1 hour or 2 will not make a difference in the results. If you continue stretching out your eating times and shortening your fasting times, look at another plan. Intermittent fasting works when you choose a plan and stick to it.

2.3 STICK WITH AN EATING PLAN FOR AT LEAST A MONTH

It is a good idea to stick with a fasting method for at least a month to see how it works for you. It will take that long for your body to get used to this new way of eating. If you do not feel it is working for you or it is too difficult to sustain, then simply try another one until you find one that you feel good with.

2.4 PLAN YOUR MEALS

Meal planning is a great way to make sure that you are getting enough calories and making sure that your body is getting the vitamins and minerals. You can make sure that you have the food you need for the week to avoid going to the grocery store. This can be highly beneficial, especially when you are going through your fasting period. When you eat, you want to make sure to eat foods that are filling yet low in calories.

There are many different ways to prepare your meals; you can do them on the weekend for the entire week or do them the night before.

Meal prepping does not have to be difficult and time-consuming. There are many ways to cut your time in half.

When you can make larger batches of the food you are going to use, it is beneficial. Sometimes I will make a family pack of chicken, then freeze what I do not use. Then I am already ahead for the following week.

2.5 TRACK YOUR CALORIES

Make sure to track your calories. Having an app to keep track of calories is much easier than trying to do it all yourself. It is simple to let them get away from you, especially when fasting. You may believe you deserve a reward for all of your hours of hard work and end up overeating and destroying your hard work. You deserve a reward but find another type of reward, like going for a walk in nature, going to the beach, getting a massage, or whatever preferred way you Like to treat yourself.

2.6 EAT HEALTHY FOODS

Whether you are fasting or feasting, steer clear of drinks with artificial flavoring and juices. Fruit juices sound like they would be healthy since they have the word fruit in them. Look at the label; they are full of sugar, carbohydrates and contain very little fruit juice.

While there are no foods that you can not eat but If you want to lose weight or become healthier, it is essential to eat healthy foods. Eating healthy does not have to be strict or be hard; simply make sure there is a balance.

You want to avoid binging on foods with high sugar content, like ice cream, soda, and similar things. Instead, you should eat plenty of vegetables, a diet high in fiber, fruits and proteins, and complex carbs. All of these will help you to feel fuller longer. It can not be said enough to drink a lot of fluids, especially water.

When coming off a fast, you may want just to sit down and start eating whatever you can. Do not do this. Make sure you are eating a meal that is healthy and full of the nutrients that you need. Eat slow and steady, chewing each piece to allow your body to start digesting it.

Unlike what we were taught in school, it is okay to skip breakfast. You can have your first meal of the day whenever you want within your fasting window. Studies from the National Center of Biotechnologies have shown you do not have to eat 2-3 snacks a day. Not eating breakfast or missing snacks do not affect keeping your metabolism functioning at an optimal level.

2.7 EAT A LOT OF FRUITS AND VEGETABLES

Make sure you are eating a lot of fruits and vegetables. The majority of your nutrients come from them; If you believe you are not getting enough, get some vitamins or take supplements; they will help ensure you are getting plenty.

The good news about fruits and vegetables is you can eat more of them, and they will have fewer calories than a single piece of chicken.

Healthy eating is not as complicated as we were taught. Eat as many whole foods as you are able and steer clear of anything processed. I have often heard the advice of adding a lot of different colors to your plate. I like this idea. After all, it looks appealing because it has a lot of nutrients packed in there.

2.8 DRINK PLENTY OF WATER

If you get hungry during your fasting time, drink some water; if that does not help, think about how much you are eating during your eating time. You may need to add more calories or add more fats and protein. The primary way to determine how fasting is working is how you feel, how you are sleeping, and how your energy is. A mistake many people make is not drinking enough water.

2.9 PROTEINS ARE VITAL

Protein is vital for IF. Proteins help to keep you full for more extended amounts of time, and they keep your muscles healthy. If you do not eat enough, you may find yourself getting hungry before your fasting ends and losing muscle mass.

To keep your muscles healthy, you need to make sure you are eating enough. One thing I do is make sure I drink a protein shake close to the end of my eating time.

Not only does the shake contain protein it also contains fiber. Both of these are great at helping to keep you full for more extended amounts of time. That and it helps you reach your recommended daily amounts.

2.10 DEAL WITH UNHEALTHY EMOTIONS

We all have different experiences growing up, and if we grew up in a home that was not focused on healthy eating, chances are we were not either. I never saw fresh fruit in my house, but I occasionally grabbed it off the tree in my front yard. As a result, I did not realize that it was customary to have fruits and vegetables available for snacks for many years. Sometimes remembering to keep fresh fruit out even now is difficult.

Many times people use eating as a way to avoid emotions. Suppose this is something that you tend to do; be prepared to have these emotions come up. One of the best things you can do when this happens is just sitting with the feeling until it passes. You can also journal about what is coming up too. This may help you to heal some things you were unaware of.

Some people are addicted to food; if you make sure, you get help for your addiction before you begin intermittent fasting.

2.11 STAY BUSY DURING PERIODS OF FASTING

During the times you are fasting, make sure to stay busy. Find things that keep your mind occupied, so there is no time to think about food. One of the advantages of fasting late is that you are sleeping most of the time during your fasting times.

Try to avoid watching too much television. This may sound like a weird idea but think about it. How many times have you sat in front of the television mindlessly snacking? The National Library of Medicine studied watching tv, and a snacking study showed that one of the primary reasons for weight gain in America is watching too much tv. When you are watching television, you are not paying attention to what you are eating and instead just putting the food in your mouth most of the time without paying attention to what it is.

2.12 DO NOT STOP EXERCISING

Many people want to lose weight with IF, and it is an excellent way too, but you do not want to do this by losing muscle mass. Muscle weighs more than fat, and frequently with this eating plan, you will notice your body changing even if your weight isn't. This may be because you are gaining muscle. You want to gain muscle, so if you see the scale creeping up, look at the changes in your body.

Do not stop working out. In the first few days, you want to do an easy workout, maybe some light walking or whatever feels good at the time, but do something. First, decide when you are going to exercise. Will you be doing it before fasting or after fasting? According to Chelsea Amengual, MS, RD. The manager of Fitness Programming and Nutrition at Virtual Health Partners suggests that exercising right after fasting will help to burn more calories. Exercising at the end of a fast may be pretty tricky since you will already be tired and not energetic.

2.13 MAKE SURE YOU ARE GETTING A GOOD NIGHT'S SLEEP

Sleep is essential when fasting. Sleeping well benefits you in many ways, similar to fasting. Healthy sleeping habits are linked to eating fewer calories during the day. You lower your chances of heart disease when you get regular sleep. People who do not sleep well have an increased risk of stroke and type 2 diabetes.

2.14 TRACK YOUR RESULTS

Keep track of your results. There are apps out there to help you keep track. On days when it is challenging to keep going, you can look back at how far you have come and stay on track. Keep a log of what you eat, when you eat, and how you feel after that. By doing this, you are going to see what works for you and what does not.

I like tracking how I feel after that. This helped me to discover many things about my body. I know that if I eat heavy foods, I quickly get bloated. I have to watch how much broccoli I eat, which is problematic because it is my favorite vegetable. I found this very helpful when I first started fasting. It was really insightful to reflect on how much I have changed and grew since beginning this journey.

2.15 SET REALISTIC EXPECTATIONS

Set realistic expectations. You are not going to lose a lot of weight weekly. This is not going to happen in 1-2 weeks because it takes time. Remember, this is not a diet plan; this is a healthy eating plan that helps you to live a longer and healthier life. I look at how it took me time to gain weight on an unhealthy diet, so it is going to take time to change the way I eat now. This is a journey, not a race. Instead of setting up a specific goal, pay attention to what you have already accomplished and how much healthier you are.

2.16 FIND A PARTNER TO WORK THE PLAN WITH

Another tip about IF if one of your friends, family member, or co-worker is doing it, talk about being accountability partners. When you first start an exercise plan, it is much easier with someone to keep you on track. When you begin different types of diets, it is easier when you have someone to cheer you on. It is the same with IF; when things get hard, you will have someone to call, and so will they. Another good part of this is you may even make a new friend.

3

Get Ready for Intermittent Fasting

3.1 GET READY FOR INTERMITTENT FASTING

This needs to be repeated; if you have any medical conditions or a woman, please get your doctor's permission before starting any new diet. Changing diets suddenly can cause a woman's hormones to fluctuate, which can cause issues. Pregnant women should also consult a physician; women need to get enough nutrients to support their babies' health. Also, if you have diabetes, make sure to check with your doctor. If you have any type of eating disorder, this may not be the diet for you.

3.1.1 BREAK DOWN INTERMITTENT FASTING INTO STEPS

According to Abigail Roaquin, BSN, RN, you should break IF down into steps before deciding if this lifestyle change is for you. There are significant benefits to Intermittent fasting. Try it for 6 months or so, observe your emotions, and watch how you feel physically. It is also important to note that you may want to allow your body to adjust if you just started exercising.

3.1.2 IDENTIFY WHAT YOUR GOALS ARE WITH THIS EATING PLAN

Most of the time, people who start IF have a specific goal in mind. Your goal could be to lose weight, work towards getting healthy, or you may want to improve your overall health. Your reason for starting Intermittent fasting will help you choose the type of eating plan you want to begin.

3.1.3 THE MENTAL PREPARATION FOR INTERMITTENT FASTING IS AS CHALLENGING AS THE PHYSICAL PREPARATION

Changing eating habits may be one of the most challenging things we do. We have been conditioned since childhood how we should eat. One essential thing to remember does not have a cheat day. If you do, you will have a tough time getting back into the flow of fasting.

The way unhealthy food affects our brain is fascinating. Maybe you drink alcohol a few times a week or love eating fast food or even at restaurants. It is easy just to grab and go with people's busy lifestyles. Making a habit of eating fast food causes you to become more impatient.

A team of Toronto researchers did a study where the researchers showed people fast food logos, then given a passage to read; the people who were shown the logos rushed through the reading of the passage.

According to the National Library of Medicine, when you eat unhealthy food, mentally, you are prone to depression. Those who ate out more frequently had an increase in depressive symptoms.

Most people in the United States have a diet that a lot of carbohydrates in it. According to the Holistic Psychologist, carbs trigger more hunger which causes you to eat more, and you end up eating every 2 hours. This is the opposite of what you want to do on the intermittent fasting plan. One step you should take is to start eating a low-carb diet before starting intermittent fasting. Instead of filling up on carbs, switch to eating foods that are higher in fats and proteins. You can also experiment with different types of low-carb diets you can explore.

When you first stop eating fewer carbs, you will experience withdrawal symptoms and many sugar cravings. With the withdrawal symptoms, be prepared to be moody and cranky. You can do a few things to help with sugar cravings, like stopping all carbs at once. Do not just ease off a little at a time because it makes it more difficult. Avoid all types of sweeteners, even stevia. While this is a better choice than refined sugar, it can still lead to more cravings. You just have to power through it.

Instead of grabbing fast food a few times a week, make meals at the beginning of the week so you will have something ready for those long days.

3.1.4 STOP EATING LATE AT NIGHT

This is difficult for some people; I know it was for me. Most people do not eat healthy late at night but instead go for cookies, ice cream, or other foods that have many high in calories and unhealthy.

According to Psychology Today, we tend to eat later at night because after avoiding temptation all day, our willpower is running low, making it easier to give in to late-night eating. Another reason late-night snacking occurs is due to the scarcity of food when our ancestors were around. Food was not as plentiful then, meaning they needed to eat as much as they were able in case there was nothing available in the morning.

3.1.5 ONCE YOU STOP EATING AT NIGHT, CHOOSE A FASTING PLAN

I went over various eating plans in chapter 1. If you need to refresh your memory, you can go back and re-read the chapter. There is Eat Stop Eat, Warrior Diet, Alternate Day Fasting, 5:2 method, 16:8 method, 14:10 method, and spontaneous meal skipping.

You now decide to try out skipping a meal and then try fasting either at 14:10 (14-hour fasting and 10-hour feasting). Another plan you may be able to start is overnight fasting. The majority of the time, you will be asleep with this fasting, making it more manageable. If any of these plans work, you can stay there; if you want more of a challenge, you can continue trying out the other ones.

Just make sure you choose the one that works best for you. One way to help you choose the best eating plan is to take a look at your lifestyle. Do you get up early and want breakfast as soon as you wake up? If so, make sure to choose a plan that will always have breakfast early. If you are a night owl, you want to start eating later in the day. You will need an eating plan where you can eat from noon-8 or later.

Doing alternate-day fasting is no more effective than doing the 16:8 or 14:10 eating plans. Doing the 24 hour fast is more likely to add to overeating, leading to weight gain. Jama Network did a study that showed that focusing on the number of calories you eat is more beneficial than fasting for 24 hours.

If you are doing alternate day fasting or the 5:2 method, do not fast for 2 consecutive days. Choose the weekdays to fast instead of the weekends. Weekdays are more structured than the weekends. In addition to having less structure, you will also have more choices in what you eat.

3.1.6 EXPECT THERE TO BE THINGS YOU HAVE TO WORK AROUND IN YOUR LIFE

This is something to remember when choosing which fasting plan is right for you. Do you like to go out for dinner occasionally? Then select the program where you are allocated eating time later in the day.

Is one of your favorite things to do is going out with some friends, having a few drinks, and eating? If this is the case, you will have to either find something else you can do as a group or do not hang out until your willpower is stronger.

3.1.7 HOW YOUR LIFESTYLE AFFECTS THE NUMBER OF CALORIES YOU NEED

If you are unsure how to figure out the number of calories and nutrients, you need to consult a dietitian.

Figuring out calories and nutrients is challenging. You can look online to do it, but I would ask a dietitian unless you have experience with it. According to Check Your Health, you can figure out the number of calories you need daily in a few different ways.

The 2 ways to do this are:

Calculate your basal metabolic rate

The Basal Metabolic Rate (BMR) is when you figure out how many calories you need when you are active versus inactive.

Physical activity - how active you really are

- Do you spend most of your day sitting? If so, you are not active.

- Do you do light activities a few times a week? An example of this would be a nice walk outside with your pet.

- If you do physical activities 2-3 times a week, like speed walking or jogging, you fall into the moderately active category.

- If you work out hard during the week, you fall into the hard exercise category. This is for people who are typically into some type of physical training, such as for a marathon.

- Extra active is for those who train or play professional sports or bodybuilding. Significantly few people fall into this category.

3.1.8 BE PREPARED FOR SIDE EFFECTS

There are a few different side effects that you need to be prepared for. The first few days, it is normal to feel both mentally and physically tired. After a week or so, you will start feeling better and have more energy.

For the first week, it will be challenging to exercise. This is normal, so do what you can and be easy on yourself. One thing to keep in mind when you plan your workouts while fasting, your body goes into metabolic stress and uses fat instead of sugar for energy, similar to what happens during the Keto diet.

3.1. 9 PLAN WAYS TO DEAL WITH STRESS

Plan ways to avoid stress. According to the American Psychological Association, stressed people are more likely to overeat and typically choose high-calorie and high-fat foods. When you are stressed, your body stores more fat than when you are in a relaxed state. Not to mention you will not feel well after binging on sugar and fat.

Another effect of stress is having trouble sleeping. This is counterproductive for intermittent fasting since sleep is such a vital part of this eating plan. Plan ways before you start intermittent fasting on how you are going to handle stress. Sutter Health wrote an article called "10 Simple Ways to Cope with Stress." One of these ways is to start a hobby. Hobbies are great ways to relax and take your mind off of things. One thing I recommend is meditation and yoga. These are also really great when you first start fasting.

There are times it is going to be hard to overcome your food cravings, and meditation can take your mind off of it. Yoga is an excellent and gentle exercise; it helps you to release tension in your body. If you have a pet to overcome, spend more time with it. Pets are a fantastic way to relieve stress and lower your blood pressure.

3.3.10 PLAN FOR THIS TO BE A LIFESTYLE CHANGE

Be prepared to make a long-term lifestyle change. Intermittent fasting is not only healthy; it also helps to simplify your life. This occurs because you spend less time cooking and more time focusing on other things. You stop constantly craving food and thinking about what you will eat later. This alone may give you extra time to look into starting a hobby. Not only is fasting good for weight loss, but it is also a fantastic way to live. Another great thing about IF is that your focus will improve along with your disciple. You will also become more productive, and we can all use that. You will become healthier, have more energy, plus you may delay chronic disease.

If you are finding this book helpful, please leave a review on Amazon.

4

How to Stay Motivated

4.1 HOW TO STAY MOTIVATED AND AVOID FEELING FRUSTRATED

When we make any lifestyle change, it's easy to become frustrated. You are not eating the way you usually do. You have changed your diet and are no longer eating the foods you want to. It makes sense all these changes can cause frustration and mood changes.

How many times have you decided this time you are going to get healthy? Nothing is going to stop you now. About a month later, you are frustrated and have lost all motivation, and are back where you started. This is not because you are failing at the diet. This happens because you have put so much pressure on yourself to be perfect. You do not know how to handle days when you feel frustrated, you have no motivation, or when you have a craving that just will not go away.

When you first get up, start drinking water

Frequently thirst masks itself as hunger, and it is difficult to tell the difference. This is especially true on days you fast. You need to go back to chapter 2 and read the tips and tricks for fasting.

Chew gum when you start feeling hungry

Make sure you choose sugar-free gum. Eating food and chewing gum both have the chewing motion tricking your body into thinking it is eating.

Call a friend

Talking to someone going through the same thing as you help to make you feel less alone. Your fasting partner will be able to identify with you and offer suggestions on how she handles the hunger.

Drink Apple Cider Vinegar

Drinking 1-2 teaspoons can help to ward off hunger, plus it absorbs minerals from meals. This absorption can help you to feel fuller for more extended amounts of time.

Stay away from food

When you are fasting, do not watch food videos, go into the kitchen or go grocery shopping. Going into the grocery store may cause you to purchase food that is not a healthy choice. Being around all of this food, whether by video or not, will be a temptation that will make it hard to stick to fasting. Science Daily researched and found that just seeing pictures of food can cause an individual to feel hungry.

Stay busy

Do not sit around watching to clock tick by. Instead, do something. If you have been putting off reading a book, do it now. Go for walks or start a hobby. There is almost always something you can do to keep busy. Frontiers in Psychology discovered that eating food is a way for people to ignore feelings of boredom.

Accept you are going to feel hungry

Of course, you are going to be hungry when not eating for long periods. Be aware that there are things that you can do to help with the hunger and do them.

Drink coffee

Coffee helps to help you feel more fuller for a more extended amount of time. Decaf coffee works slightly better than caffeinated kind.

Avoid alcohol

Alcohol contains a lot of carbohydrates which will make you hungrier.

Go to bed early

This is one of the easiest ways to help you feel full. Sleep your fasting time away.

When we are at work, we will start to feel hungry and head to the vending machine

Instead of doing that, bring healthy snacks with you that can help tide you over. I like having a trail mix with different nuts and fruits inside it, but there are all sorts of healthy snacks you can choose from. One I love is cucumbers; if I know I am going to be out running around for a while, I will cut up some cucumbers and put them in a container within a cooler, and they not only provide a healthy snack, they are very hydrating.

- You can go through periods of depression when starting your new healthy lifestyle. According to VIVEVE, chocolate releases serotonin in your brain, which creates a feeling of happiness. The good news is that fruits naturally have these nutrients in them also.

- The Indian Journal of Psychiatry did a study in 2008 that showed that our choice of food affects depression. Frequently people believe that depression is based on brain chemicals or emotions. The research mentioned above indicates that healthy eating and good food choices can help with the severity and/or length of depressive symptoms.

- Like many substances, sugar and processed foods are addicting. You will have headaches; you will be tired and cranky for a few days. Foods that are high in sugar and fats make you feel energy instantly; the bad news about that is that you have the sugar crash shortly after. Healthy foods do not cause instant energy instead it gradually increases energy after time.

- You need to make sure you are eating enough calories from the right foods. You need to eat roughly 1,350 calories on the days you are not fasting.

- Making sure you have enough omega-3 fatty acids helps to keep you motivated when eating healthy. There are many benefits to making sure you get enough omegas in your diet; it is vital for mentally healthy and brain health as well as helping to maintain blood sugar.

- Get rid of temptation lurking in your home. If you have a lot of unhealthy food in your home, you are going to want it. Clear your food from all of these temptations. If you have a family who enjoys these types of foods, cleaning out the cupboards will help them eat better. Instead of junk food, stock up on yogurt and fresh berries. I have also heard that replacing potato chips with baked provolone cheese helps with the cravings.

- Pay attention to self-talk. Are you constantly thinking negative things about yourself or putting yourself down? These negative thoughts can lead to a loss of motivation. When that happens, do your best to put a stop to it. Tell yourself what a fantastic job you have been doing and how proud you are. If needed, put encouraging phrases through your house. I am strong; I am winning, I am healthy, I have come a long way, etc.

- On days you feel low, call a friend to see if they want to do something together like going to the gym, swimming, or playing tennis.

4.1.3 I AM SO TIRED OF COUNTING CALORIES

- Some foods that are considered healthy are high in calories; a perfect example of this is an avocado which has roughly 300 calories. Healthy food that is packed with vitamins and minerals can be high in calories. So while calorie counting is good, make sure to consider its benefits too.

- Studies have shown that when you lower your calories all at once, it leaves you feeling frustrated and exhausted. It is challenging to stay motivated to live a healthy lifestyle if you are constantly hungry and in a bad mood. One way to help alleviate this side effect is to cut back slowly instead of all at once.

- Tracking calories is not a way to control your behavior; instead, it allows you to study it.

- Do not worry about being perfect. It is nearly impossible to get the correct number of calories on the dot.

- Worry more about the quality of calories instead of quantity. If you ate 2 cups of spinach and thought you ate 1 cup, that is far better than eating 6 cookies and thinking you ate only 3.

- When in doubt, get an app. There are excellent calorie counting apps out there; just pick one.

4.1.4 I AM SO TIRED OF FEELING TIRED

- Starting a healthy lifestyle is tiring; it feels like you are consistently planning out healthy meals, deciding on what snacks are the best, fighting temptation constantly, and finding time to work out. You can take a break. You do not have to plan all the time and exercise daily. Just grab a salad for dinner one night or something healthy that is already in your fridge. If you work out too often or hard, you can hurt yourself and put off your weight loss goals. Remember, life is meant to be fun and not always about planning.

- Get outside and take a 15-minutes walk to get out of the slump on those rough days. Oddly, you will feel more energy if you get up and do something.

- If you need extra motivation or other ideas, go back and read chapters 2 and 3.

4.1.5. I AM FRUSTRATED ALL THE TIME

- Do some cardio or weight lifting for about 30 minutes. Exercise is one of the best ways to get endorphins going, lower stress, and improve your mood. One thing to remember is when you exercise or weight lift for over 1 hour, it can leave you in a worse mood than when you started, plus cause you to feel drained.

- Get a fitness tracker or something similar. When I look down and see how many steps I have taken or how many calories I have burned during the day, it makes me want to keep working.

- Go outside. Healthy exercise is not just working out at a gym or aerobics in front of the television; there are many other types. Go for a hike, go to a beach, get outdoors and do something fun. This will keep your mood up and give you time just to relax.

- Remember, as we age, our metabolism slows down. We are no longer 20 where you can eat an entire cake and walk for 10 minutes without affecting your body. Unless you are one of the lucky ones who can still do that, accepting that our body no longer metabolizes food as it used to is something to remember when we feel the scale is not going down quick enough or those jeans are not as loose as they should be.

- Lifestyle changes are not as easy as you expected. According to the European Journal of Social Psychology, it can take around 66 days to adjust to a healthy lifestyle. In time making healthy choices will become as simple as tying your shoes.

- On days you are frustrated, are you overthinking about foods that you no longer eat? You may be restricting yourself too much. When you limit yourself too much, you may end up binge eating. Let yourself have a small portion of your favorite treat occasionally. This is much better than ruining all you have worked for.

4.1.6. I FEEL LIKE GIVING UP

- Take pictures every week to see the progress you have made; that's always an excellent way to keep up motivation. I love looking back to see how far I have come. Not just in regards to weight loss but also overall. Just think how good it feels when you go in for a checkup, and your doctor says you are in excellent health.

- Why did you decide to start eating healthy? What are the benefits you get from healthy eating? If you have been keeping track of your journey, reading can show you how far you have come.

- Practice gratitude even to yourself. Just being thankful for what you have accomplished is enough. Yesterday you did not eat that cheeseburger you wanted so much. Today you walked by that cake and said no. You are amazing; what a good job you are doing.

- Take a look at your fasting partner. How is she doing? Use her as inspiration to keep going too.

- Take it one day at a time. Do not look ahead to a few years from now; focus only on today.

- Create a smaller goal and obtain it. Write a blog, learn a new healthy recipe and then have friends over for dinner. Walk the extra mile. If you do one of these, you will feel much better.

- Figure out why you want to give up once you discover the answer, find out how to fix it. Maybe you feel like you need another hour of eating. Change your plan up a bit.

5

Detailed Plans On How to Start a Healthy Lifestyle in 14 Days

5.1 PLAN 1 FOR A HEALTHIER LIFESTYLE

Fasting sounds like a great idea to get healthy, but what do I eat? What kind of exercises do I do? And what does the fast actually look like?

Below I will show you the fasting plan 14:10. This is where you fast for 14 hours and then eat for 10 hours. This is a great plan to start because most of your fasting time will be happening while you sleep. The easiest way to do this plan is to fast from 7 P.M. to 9 A.M. then eat from 9 A.M. to 7 P.M.

You can always rearrange this schedule to what best fits your schedule. I know some people have different work schedules that may make this eating schedule difficult.

Each day I will give you different physical activities to do, some include exercises, and others are more relaxing. There are 3 meals and daily snacks included in this daily plan, along with some vital tips to keep in mind. If you eat during your fasting time, do not get discouraged; if you overindulge during your eating time, do not get down on yourself. You can just pick up right where you left off. Chocolate is something I love; I can happily eat it daily. I know for a healthy lifestyle, I can't do this, but I can have a single square of dark chocolate twice a month.

5.1.1 WEEK 1

Welcome to the first week of the rest of your life. I am here to help you step by step through working the 14:10 intermittent plan.

)THE 14:10 DIET

	DAY 1	DAY 2	DAY 3	DAY 4	DAY 5	DAY 6	DAY 7
MIDNIGHT 4 AM	FAST	FAST	FAST	FAST	FAST	FAST	FAST
10 AM 12 PM	First meal	First meal	First meal	First meal	First meal	First meal	First meal
4 PM	Last meal by 8PM	Last meal by 8PM	Last meal by 8PM	Last meal by 8PM	Last meal by 8PM	Last meal by 8PM	Last meal by 8PM
8 PM MIDNIGHT	FAST	FAST	FAST	FAST	FAST	FAST	FAST

Week 1 grocery list

- 2 Avocados
- 2 Garlic Cloves
- 2 Lemons
- 2 Oranges
- 2 Oranges
- 3 Green Bell Peppers
- Apples
- Asparagus

- Bacon
- Banana
- Blueberries
- Brussel Sprouts
- Carrots
- Caster Sugar
- Cheddar Cheese
- Cherry Tomatoes

- Chia Seeds
- Chicken
- Chicken Burger
- Chili
- Chili Flakes
- Chives
- Chopped Romaine
- Coriander

- Cottage Cheese
- Cream Cheese
- Cucumbers
- Cumin Seeds
- Dijon Mustard
- Eggs
- English Cucumber
- Feta Cheese
- Feta Cheese Crumbled
- Fish Sauce
- Frozen Shelled Edamame
- Ginger
- Greek Yogurt
- Hot Vegetable Stock Cubes
- Hummus
- Italian Seasoning
- Kale
- Kiwi
- Lime
- Lime
- Mango
- Mayonnaise
- Milk
- Milk
- Muesli
- Naan Bread
- Olive Oil
- Onion
- Peanut Butter
- Pear
- Pepper
- Portobello Mushroom
- Red Lentil
- Red Onion
- Red Wine Vinegar
- Ricotta Cheese
- Roquefort Cheese
- Salad Greens
- Salmon
- Salt
- Shallots
- Spinach
- Sriracha
- Tilapia
- Toasted Sesame Oil
- Tomato
- Tomatoes
- White Beans
- Yogurt

Day 1

While there is no rule about what time to eat and what to eat, I will refer to the first meal of the day as your morning meal. For this, have a healthy green smoothie. These are loaded with nutrients to help get your body moving. Try to eat within 1 hour or so when you break your fast. This will allow you not to overindulge later in the day; if you are used to exercising, start with your everyday exercise. I like doing HIIT workouts once a week, 1 day of Interval training, and 3 days of lifting weights. Then twice a week I take walks or do something fun with friends. For your first day, do weight lifting, just to find out where you are. When I first started, I put no weights on my bars.

At noon for lunch, have a Cobb salad with vinaigrette dressing. Make sure to make your own dressing; otherwise, there will be many additives that you do not need in your body. Vinaigrette dressing is so easy to make; you simply need oil, vinegar, and seasoning. I use balsamic vinegar because I love it, but you can use whatever you prefer. For an activity, after lunch, it is nice just to get outside and take your dogs for a walk or just walk around and enjoy nature.

I like something simple in the afternoon, a piece of fruit paired with a type of dip. Apple and 2 tablespoons of peanut butter is excellent and will get you through the afternoon hump. Make sure you are staying hydrated. It is essential to make sure you are using all-natural peanut butter. Pay attention to the label because some that claim to be all-natural are not. For an easy activity after your snack, you can try out gardening. Anytime you are unmotivated, look back in chapter 4 to get back on the right path.

Dinner is a great time just to sit back and relax. Tonight, for dinner, I would suggest a serving of sheet pan chicken with Brussel sprouts. A good tip is to make extra chicken and Brussel sprouts so you can freeze them and eat them later in the week. Cooked chicken is good frozen for up to four months. If it is covered with broth, it can last up to 6 months. Since it is close to bedtime, it is good to end your day with something relaxing like yoga.

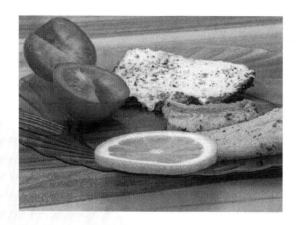

Day 2

For a healthy breakfast this morning, you can have an omelet with Feta cheese and spinach. Remember, you want natural cheese that is not processed. For your physical activity today, grab some weights and start lifting. If you are a beginner, make sure to start with lighter weights that you feel comfortable using. For lunch, an apple kale wrap and chicken would taste great and has the protein you need. Make sure you are paying attention to serving sizes. Today you can try gardening for a bit. If you do not garden already, it is a great hobby to start. Remember, fresh is best when eating kale. For the afternoon snack, an orange with 20 almonds is excellent and full of healthy fats and nutrients. Make sure your almonds are unsalted to avoid extra sodium. In the afternoon, it is the perfect time to go outside for a walk. For dinner, baked salmon with asparagus. Asparagus has always been one of my favorite vegetables, even though my family disagrees. For the evening activity, try out meditation. Get a good night's sleep; it is vital for the mind and body.

Day 3

For your first meal, have 1 cup of plain Greek yogurt, 1 cup of blueberries, and 1/3 cup of muesli. Some manufacturers try to sneak in added sugar in the muesli; make sure to check the label. Interval training is a great morning activity. If you have not done it before, make sure you start with a beginner one. For lunch, white bean and vegetable salad would be a good choice. If you have any vinaigrette left, this is the perfect chance to use it. Save some white beans for another day. Walking is an excellent activity after lunch. It gives your body a chance to use some of the energy. Another afternoon snack I enjoy is a bell pepper cut into strips with a tablespoon of cream cheese; you can switch the cream cheese out for hummus if you prefer. A good tip to remember for lunch is to cut up extra green peppers for another day. Green peppers can last 2-3 days when wrapped in a paper towel and stored in a ziplock bag. For an excellent afternoon activity gardening. For dinner, a Greek salad with edamame sounds excellent. A good dressing to go with Greek salad is simply called Greek salad dressing, and again it is super easy to make. 1 clove of garlic, olive oil, red wine vinegar, some lemon juice, dijon mustard, dried oregano, salt, and pepper. Many of these items you probably already have in your home. Make sure not to eat processed food. They are terrible for you and do not taste well at all. Tonight before bed, try some relaxing yoga.

Day 4

For your first meal of the day, how about a spinach and Feta cheese omelet? Make sure you have fresh spinach and cheese that is not processed. For your first morning activity, do some weight lifting. This will help you to gain muscle mass and burn more calories.

For lunch, have a Portobello chicken burger with Feta and shallots. It is always a good thing to save any extra that you have to use again. After lifting weights this morning, a nice long walk would be nice to loosen some of the muscles you just used. Need more tips? Look back in chapter 3 for some reminders.For the afternoon snack, have a hard-boiled egg with Cheddar cheese. If you boil multiple eggs, you can always use them as a quick snack or even for breakfast if you do not feel like cooking. This would be a lovely time of the day to get outside and garden.

For dinner, have a serving of spiced carrot and lentil soup. Freeze what is leftover to pair with a salad later in the week. A good activity for this time of the day would be meditation. It's always good to end your day with something relaxing.

Day 5

An excellent way to break your fast is with a healthy banana smoothie. You can make smoothies and freeze them. Just make sure to put them in your refrigerator the night before you want to drink them so they can thaw out. When you make your smoothies, make sure not to use fruit juice. You can add plain Greek yogurt to it, milk, non-dairy milk if you have milk allergies or are lactose intolerant. Today is another day of interval training.Today for lunch, Asian chicken salad with sesame ginger dressing. Make extra dressing so you can save some. Make sure to make an extra serving of the salad so you can have it for dinner tonight. After interval training this morning, you want to do something more relaxing, like hanging out with a friend.

For the afternoon, a kiwi and mango smoothie. Instead of doing something physical tonight, why not just meditate. It is a great way to relax and release any stress of the day. Make sure each night you are taking a warm shower or bath to keep your muscles relaxed. Here is when you can use the rest of your Asian chicken salad paired with garlic lemon-baked tilapia. After dinner, if it is dark, you can take a nice walk under the stars; if it lights out still, then go out and enjoy some sun. If you add lemon to your tilapia, it will bring out the flavor.

Day 6

How about avocado egg toast this morning for your first meal? Then head outside to do some jogging. If you are not up for jogging, try speed walking. It is essential to mix up your exercises not to get bored, and your body does not adapt to the same ones.

For lunch, spiced carrot and lentil soup sound good. As always, freeze some for another meal. It is always nice to have some extra meals frozen to grab them when you do not feel like cooking. If you have excess to a pool, take a break and go for a nice swim. Many gyms have indoor pools, and if not, most hotels have one they will let you pay for so you can swim. After a swim, you will probably be ready for a snack; how about 1 medium pear with a serving of cottage cheese? If you have an extra pear, keep it on hand for lunch on the day after your afternoon snack; take a nice walk to let your food settle. For dinner, let's have a serving of Acquacotta. I came across this recipe, and it looked amazing, so I had to share it. It is eggplant tomato soup with a lot of vegetables. A good tip for this soup is to make extra so that you can have it another night. It is just that good. Tonight before bed, do some yoga. So you will be ready for your next day of fasting.

Day 7

This is your final day of fasting for this week. Like each night, go to bed early and enjoy a good night's sleep. In the morning, start your day off with Ricotta, tomato, and spinach frittata. For your first morning activity, go outside and put your hands in some dirt by gardening. A little-known fact is when you are digging or gardening, it improves your immune system and relaxes you. At noon set down and have something to drink with your white bean and veggie salad. Today is a great day to go out with a friend and play a few games of tennis. Hanging out with a friend is always a good idea because socializing is essential. You have made it to the afternoon. Have a simple medium orange for today's snack. Oranges are simple snacks that are refreshing. I am a fan of mandarin oranges. They are my favorite. After that, go out and have a relaxing walk; even 20 minutes is enough to feel better. For evening, chicken vegetable fajita — use your leftover green peppers and spinach here. Instead of using typical wraps for the fajita, you can make one called dosa. Tonight after your bath or shower, do some yoga before bed. Pat yourself on the back and do something special as a reward. You just made it through your first week.

The 14:10 fasting is a great way to start when you begin fasting. If you want to go for long hours of fasting, you can simply increase your fasting times by 1 hour until you reach your desired fasting time.

5.1.2 WEEK 2
Week 2 grocery list

- Asparagus
- Avocado
- Banana
- Black Beans
- Blackberries
- Blueberries
- Broccoli
- Carrots
- Celery
- Cheddar Cheese
- Chicken
- Cinnamon
- Coconut
- Cranberries
- Cucumbers
- Eggs
- Feta
- Flax Seed
- Garlic
- Ginger
- Goat Cheese
- Green Peppers
- Ham
- Honeydew Melon
- Kale
- Masala
- Medallions
- Mozzarella Cheese
- Mushrooms
- Onions
- Orange Pepper
- Parmesan
- Pepperoni
- Pork Chop
- Portobello Mushrooms
- Potatoes
- Raspberries
- Raspberry Vinaigrette
- Red Pepper
- Rice
- Romaine Lettuce
- Salad Greens
- Salmon
- Sauce
- Sausage
- Shallots
- Sherry Vinegar
- Spinach
- Sprouted Grain Bread
- Strawberries
- Sweet Potato
- Tilapia
- Turkey
- Vegetable Broth
- Yellow Pepper
- Yogurt
- Zucchini

Day 8

This morning how about a ham, Mozzarella cheese, and mushroom omelet. Omelets are always a great way to start your day. They are packed full of all the nutrients and will keep you going until lunch. Keep in mind Mozzarella cheese does not freeze well; if you have leftovers, use them in the next 2-4 days. A great way to start your week is by jumping right into weight lifting. You may be starting to lift more weight than you used to, be careful not to overdo it. Working out in the morning helps to keep your body in its natural rhythm.

One of my favorite lunches is Cobb salad with brown derby dressing. You can freeze brown derby dressing to use later. Today would be a good thing to go for a long walk and just relax. While you are walking, check in with your body just to see how you are feeling.

This afternoon for your snack, have 2 ounces Greek yogurt with 1 tablespoon of blueberries and cinnamon. The cinnamon helps to add a little flavor to your yogurt. For your afternoon activity go out and garden. I love to garden; it is such a relaxing activity. Keep resisting the urge to binge.

Tonight for dinner, have a chicken breast stuffed with Goat cheese and asparagus. A great way to end your day is to take a light night walk under the stars if the weather allows. Each day remember to do something to enjoy yourself.

Day 9

For your first meal of the day, have some scrambled eggs with Cheddar cheese and vegetables. Make sure you cut extra vegetables so you can use them later. Today start your weight lifting. Just be careful not to lift too much.

Today for lunch, have a serving of black bean soup. Some people like to add 1 tablespoon of sour cream with their black bean soup. Remember, every physical activity does not have to be difficult so remember that.

For your physical activity speed, walk for 2 miles. Make sure to save the soup for day 12 lunch.

For the afternoon snack, 1 tablespoon of honeydew melon and 1 tablespoon of cranberries or raspberries. Today for your physical activity, do some yoga. It is a great way to relax and get your mind to focus on the here and now.

Tonight for dinner, try out a club tilapia Parmesan; this is amazing and tastes great. Do not forget to eat plenty of vegetables with dinner. For your evening activity, finish your day with meditation. Meditation is a great way to relax before bed.

Day 10

Let's get our day going right with a delicious green kale smoothie with flax seed and strawberries thrown in. I read an article the other day that said to make sure you only eat organic strawberries. After breakfast, head out for a morning jog, or you can do speed walking if you are not up to jogging.

For lunch, have a Portobello chicken burger with Feta and shallots. As long as you mince up the shallots and place them in a ziplock bag, you can freeze them. Today why not call up a friend and go out to play badminton. No matter how well or bad you do, the laughter will be worth it. For later, something to keep in mind is if you are a fan of pizza, or rice cauliflower is a great substitute.

On day 10, If you have not started your meal plan for next week, you can start doing so now. Start by taking inventory of food you have frozen, groceries you have leftover, and what you may need for the following week's grocery list.

If you have never had pepperoni bites today, it is time to give them a try. I love these. Earlier, you had time to socialize, so why not go out to do the next best thing, gardening. If you are looking for more or fewer calories, you can add or take away from the food. An example would be at your snack time, add some almonds for a few calories. For fewer calories, you could substitute the rice in the spiced pepper pilafs for cauliflower.

To wrap up your day, have spiced pepper pilafs for dinner. After that, is the best time to do something relaxing to finish your night. Tonight would be a great night to learn something different like tai-chi. The more often you use relaxation techniques, the better you will feel.

Day 11

I love zucchini, so I think this is the perfect day for a zucchini omelet with spinach and Mozzarella cheese. After breakfast, go out and do interval training. While paying attention to your body, try to challenge yourself today.

For lunch today, try a sausage casserole with Cheddar cheese. This is great to freeze so you can eat it another day. Since you worked out this morning, you probably want to do something that is not strenuous, like going for a walk. After working out, make sure you drink a lot of water.

For your afternoon snack, enjoy half a cucumber with 1 tablespoon of ranch dressing. Cucumbers are so hydrating and healthy for you. After lunch, you can go back out and garden. You should do it every other day, if not daily, so you can keep the weeds out; plus, it is fantastic.

For dinner, have fillet medallions with blackberry, Feta, and spinach salad. Why not use some of the brown derby dressing that you froze earlier this week. After dinner, take a pleasant 30-minutes walk with a pet. If you do not have a pet, animal shelters are always looking for volunteers.

Day 12

This sounds so good for breakfast that it may become my new favorite; berry coconut breakfast parfait. After enjoying breakfast, do some more weight lifting. The nice thing about weight lifting is you can use free weights, hand weights, machines, or even your body weight.

For lunch, enjoy a serving of black bean soup. Adding sauce to your soup will give it a low-calorie zest of flavor. Find a friend to play frisbee. That would be something fun to do that you may not have done in years. Relaxing at the end of the day is vital for self-care.

A healthy snack for this afternoon is sprouted-grain toast with peanut butter and banana. I never thought I would enjoy peanut butter and banana together, but I do. After having a good snack, it would be a good time for some meditation. Prepare your breakfast tonight, so you do not have to in the morning.

For dinner, tonight, have Chicken, Quinoa, and sweet potato casserole with 2 cups of green and 1 cup of cucumber with raspberry vinaigrette. After dinner, let us switch it up a bit and try out dancing to your favorite music. If you have anyone in the house with you, make them do it with you. Make as much as you can on your own, so you do not have all the added preservatives. For example, make your sauce. I love doing this so I can experiment with different ingredients.

Day 13

I love making vegetable quiche for breakfast because you can make a lot of it to freeze, and it stays good for a long time. Our morning activity today will be speed walking or jogging. Keeping a journal on how you are feeling is great for your journey. Emotions may start coming up since you are no longer using food as a source of comfort.

For lunch, try out sauerkraut salad. Sauerkraut is such a versatile food; you can use it for many things such as soups, sauerkraut, and sausage meals. You often walk during the day, but today try out speed walking, or you can change it up a little and speed walk for a block and then walk a block to see how that feels.

Make some zucchini chips for today's afternoon snack. And while you are chopping, save a few extra for breakfast in the morning. It is a great idea to make your sauerkraut to avoid added chemicals and preservatives. Since it is later in the afternoon, go outside for a while and spend some time in your garden.

For dinner, have pork chop with sesame broccoli and save some broccoli for lunch tomorrow. For some added flavor to your water, throw in some fruit. Sometimes I like to add cucumber and lemon to mine. Tonight before bed, do some yoga to relax.

Day 14

Today is the last day of your 14-day plan, so be ready to do something great for yourself. For breakfast this morning, have vegetable frittata. Adding sauce is always good in an egg dish. After breaking you're fast, try a HIIT (High-intensity interval training), do a low-impact easy one. While the high-intensity part is usually 15-30 seconds, it is not easy.

At noon have salmon, avocado, and feta green leaf salad; if you have some vinaigrette dressing left, use it. It would make the perfect addition. It is time to start thinking about your meal plan for next week. After 30 minutes of HIIT aerobics, you will not want to do anything intense the rest of the day. At noon take it easy with a pleasant stroll. You can get the same results with interval training, where you walk fast for five minutes then walk at an average pace for 1 minute.

For today's afternoon snack, have a banana with 2 tablespoons of peanut butter. For some relaxation, take time to meditate now for at least 20 minutes. If you drift off to sleep, do not worry about it. You have had a long week and may need the added rest.

For dinner, try out some turkey stuffed green pepper with salad. You should have a few dressing left; try whichever one sounds good to you. When meditating, if you use a candle or some fragrance, it can help to relax you more. Tonight for your last activity before bed, do some yoga to help stretch out the muscles you have used today.

You have finished your 2-weeks fasting plan. How are you feeling? Did you keep a journal, so you know where you started to where you are now? There is always a sense of accomplishment when completing something you have not tried before, especially if it is something new, like being healthy. Now that you have completed this fourteen-day fast, your next one should be easier.

There are so many ways to fast; this is just one of the many options. Just times are laid out such as 14:10, 16:8, interval fasting, etc., does not mean you can not make up your own. A study was done by the University of Illinois in Chicago compared intermittent fasting times. One was a 6-hours time-restricted, and the other was a 4-hours time-restricted one. The results showed no significant differences between the 4-hour and 6-hour restricted eating fasts. This is to let you know that you do not always do the most challenging plan to make a difference. Fasting is not about eating as infrequently as you can. It is about having a healthy lifestyle.

If you are finding this book helpful, please leave a review on Amazon.

5.2.1 Week 1

The Eat-Stop-Eat fasting method is simply fasting for 24 hours twice a week. It is important to note that you do not do the 24 hour fasting period back to back. You can tailor this program to what suits you. You can fast from 8:00 P.M. to 8:00 P.M., or if you do not like that, then you can fast from 4:00 P.M. to 4:00 P.M. That's the great thing about this plan, as long as you are fasting for 24 hours you can still eat daily.

THE 5:2 DIET

DAY 1	DAY 2	DAY 3	DAY 4	DAY 5	DAY 6	DAY 7
Eats normally	Women: 500 calories Men: 600 calories	Eats normally	Eats normally	Women: 500 calories Men: 600 calories	Eats normally	Eats normally

Week 1 grocery list

- Almonds
- Banana
- Blueberries
- Celery
- Chia Seeds
- Chicken
- Chicken Broth
- Cocoa
- Cucumber
- Dijon Mustard
- Dried Black Beans
- Dried Split Peas
- Edamame
- Feta Cheese
- Green Bell Peppers
- Greens
- Ham
- Hemp Hearts

- Lemon
- Lettuce
- Mango
- Milk
- Mushrooms
- Oatmeal
- Onion
- Pork

- Chops
- Pumpkin Seeds
- Raspberries
- Salmon
- Salmon
- Spinach
- Squash
- Strawberries

- Sweet Potato
- Turkey Burger
- Unsalted Almonds
- Yogurt
- Zucchini

Day 1

Smoothies are one of the best ways to start your morning. Let's begin this morning with a blueberry smoothie. Whenever possible, use fresh blueberries. We will start your first day of this week with weight lifting. Studies have shown that weight lifting three times a week is as effective as intense cardio workouts.

A great lunch is a serving of fried kale and broccoli salad. This recipe contains mayonnaise; if you do not want to use store-bought, it is easy to make. To make mayonnaise, you simply need to combine egg yolk, vinegar, and olive oil. The color of the mayonnaise will be a brighter yellow, but that is normal. Around noon take a nice relaxing walk. Ensure you are eating enough protein during the day, or you will not find yourself being tired throughout the day.

A healthy snack during the afternoon is 1 cup of plain Greek yogurt and 1/2 cup of cucumber. You can use the yogurt as a dip. Cucumbers are a great snack because they are both hydrating and low in calories. To stay active and relax, go out and spend some time in your garden.

Here is where the broccoli you had earlier will come in handy. For dinner, try some pan-seared salmon with broccoli and cheese. I love broccoli and cheese. When I first started eating broccoli, that was how I would eat it. Now I love it boiled without anything but a bit of salt and pepper. For a tremendous nighttime activity, try out mediation. Guided meditations are fun to do.

Day 2 — fasting day

Today is the first day of your fast. You will experience hunger, but there are different tricks you can do to help with that. Today when you get up, grab a cup of coffee, tea, water, whichever you prefer. For your first morning activity, do some weight lifting. This will help you to gain muscle mass and burn more calories.

For noon, you can go with the earlier ideas of coffee, water, or tea. Herbal tea is a great way to help you feel full. This is a great time to go out for a nice relaxing walk. Walking is a great way to stay healthy and relax.

In the afternoon, drink water, coffee, or tea. You can add cinnamon to your tea to help with your hunger. A great physical activity at this time of the day is yoga. This gives your mind and body time to relax and puts a minor strain on your body.

In the evening, you can go outside and play with your dogs. You are almost done with your first fast. If you have not already, make sure you drink something. A great way to make sure you are getting enough water is a water bottle of one of those gallon jugs that come with purified water in them. Then mark how much water you need throughout the day on the jug.

Day 3

When you wake up for an excellent first meal, you can grab a handful of unsalted almonds (20 almonds is the perfect amount) and a green protein shake. Here is an example of one that would be packed with protein — Almond milk, a banana, mango, spinach, pumpkin seeds, and hemp hearts. For a morning activity, you can do some jogging. If you are not up for jogging, try speed walking.

A healthy lunch full of fiber is a serving Italian white bean soup. A great tip for this lunch is to make extra soup so you can use it for day 9; if the weather is nice, head out for a bike ride. When lifting weights, you want to do different areas: upper arms, legs, chest and back, and abs and butt. There is no rule; you can do them in whatever way you choose.

One day I went to a sushi restaurant and discovered edamame and loved it. It is such simple food and yet so filling. For today's afternoon snack, grab 1/2 cup of it. A half-hour of yoga will help you to stretch out and relax after physical activity.

A serving of vegetable curry with spiralized squash noodles is great for dinner. If you like rice with your dinner, make some cauliflower rice. Tonight is the perfect night for meditation. According to a recent study done by the Eco-Institute, doing meditation can help individuals lose 63% more weight due to being mindful.

Day 4

For breakfast, have a serving of the size of oatmeal almond protein pancakes with blueberries. The serving size of these pancakes is about 2-3 inches. After breakfast, it would be an excellent time to take a walk. Call a friend to see if they would like to join you. When you make lifestyle changes, it is always a good idea to have someone there to support you.

For lunch today, have a serving of Feta cheese stuffed with green pepper. Make some of the stuffed peppers to use another day. These are great to freeze. For a fun activity, try to hula hoop for 10 minutes. I guarantee hula hooping for just 10 minutes will cause you to sweat.

For your afternoon snack, you can use some of the green peppers you cut earlier. Today's snack, try 1/4 cup of hummus with bell pepper cut into wedges. You can save sliced green peppers for up to 12 months. After your snack, go outside and garden for a while. Even though gardening does not feel like a strenuous physical activity, your body will get sore and feel tender.

For dinner, have some grilled salmon with vegetables. Make sure to freeze any leftover vegetables to make meal preparation easier during the week. After your long busy day, take a nice warm shower or bath. If you decide to take a bath, light a candle to create a more relaxing environment.

Day 5 — fasting day

During your second fast of the week, wake up and have a black coffee, tea, or a glass of water. You can add lemon or cucumber to your water for a bit more flavor. Today's morning activity will be weight lifting. Lifting weights on your fasting day will help you build more lean muscle because your body is burning fat instead of sugar.

Around noon set down and have a glass of water, tea, or coffee; if you feel hungry, you can add some cinnamon to your tea or coffee; I am not too sure how it would taste added to water. Go outside and enjoy a nice walk. If you have dogs, take them with you. Daily exercise is great, but it is essential to pace yourself and add some gentle exercises.

When you are fasting, it is so important to make sure you are hydrated enough. This afternoon set down and have something to drink. In the afternoon, find something different without sugar to drink. Just drinking water, tea, and coffee. I have already suggested adding lemon to your water, but you can also use berries and sparkling water, and if your fasting is not too restrictive, you can have some bone broth. After your snack, do yoga for 30 minutes as a way to stretch out. A good tip is to measure yourself weekly is an excellent way to keep track of your progress.

This evening make sure you have had enough to drink throughout the day. If not, drink some more, so make sure you are hydrated. Meditation is a great thing to do before bed to relax. There is a type of meditation called Visual Meditation that is very relaxing.

Day 6

On the morning of this day, have a cocoa-chia pudding with raspberries break your fast. You can prepare this the night before or make it earlier in the week, then freeze it. You just need to remember to take it out of the freezer the night before you plan on eating it. After eating, it is an excellent time to head out for a walk. To avoid stomach issues such as gas, bloating, and other types of stomach discomfort, increase your intake of fiber slowly.

For today's lunch, enjoy a serving of Mediterranean grilled chicken salad. Make sure to save a serving for dinner. Today for something different deep clean your house. This is a good idea for two reasons you get a clean house and some great exercise.

For today's afternoon snack, try a turkey and lettuce roll-up. The serving size of this snack is considered to be 100.1 grams, plus it is full of protein. Go out and have some fun playing frisbee with a friend. When you were young, it was easy to socialize and have fun. As we age, we have to get inventive.

For dinner, have a serving of lemon Dijon pork with your leftover Mediterranean grilled chicken salad. Tonight again, do a relaxation exercise such as Tai-Chi. This is extremely gentle that increases flexibility, balance and gives your muscles definition. This exercise is so gentle that almost anyone can do it.

Day 7

For your morning meal, have a strawberry smoothie. You can make this with just 4 ingredients: strawberries, banana, yogurt, and your choice of liquid. The liquid can be anything from water to some type of milk with no sugar added. Go out and take a walk with your dog; it is nice to get outside to start your day right. It is important to remember to make sure you do some sort of activity throughout the day; it will keep your mind busy.

For today's lunch, have some split pea soup. Most soups freeze quickly for later use. Today take a few extra steps. When going out, find somewhere to park; find a spot that is farther out; when you have the chance take the steps instead of an elevator. Something as simple as where you park and choosing to take the extra steps is a way to increase your activity.

Eating 2 stalks of celery with 2 tablespoons of peanut butter is a great afternoon snack. The peanut butter will help you to feel full, while the celery will add hydration. Make sure that your peanut butter is natural. After your afternoon snack, head out to your garden. Gardening is a great way to grow your fruits and vegetables, so you will know that they are natural and healthy.

For tonight's dinner, have a sweet potato with black beans. While canned black beans may be easier to prepare, you want to buy dried black beans. Make sure when you purchase them that there are no broken beans. The package should be sealed with no holes in the bag. Holes can be a sign of bugs. This evening sit down and read a book to relax: it is a good idea to take it a little easier.

5.2.2 WEEK 2

Week 2 grocery list

- Avocado
- Bacon
- Blueberries
- Butter
- Cantaloupe
- Cauliflower
- Cheddar Cheese
- Cherry Tomatoes
- Chickpeas
- Coconut Wate
- Cucumber
- Eggs
- Farro
- Feta Cheese
- Garlic
- Garlic

- Green Onion
- Hamburger
- Kale
- Lemon

- Mixed Greens
- Mozzarella Cheese
- Nutmeg
- Olives

- Onions
- Pecans
- Portobellos
- Potatoes

Day 8 — fasting day

When you wake up, have something to drink. This is important for two reasons; first, it will wake you up and keep you hydrated, the second is that it helps you feel fuller. After your morning routine, get ready to list some weight. One of the key factors in succeeding with fasting is to make sure to keep your stress low.

Around noon you can check in with yourself to see how you are feeling. This is an excellent time to do some journaling so you can look back to see how your fasting is going. If you are really hungry, keep in mind you can eat up to 500 calories as needed. This is an excellent time to go outside with your dogs to play or take a walk. Do not drink water infused with flavors. These may sound good, but they contain artificial sweeteners, which may cause you to become hungry and overeat.

During the afternoon, you always want to make sure you are hydrating enough. Today you should take time to call a friend, read a book or take a nap. Keeping busy is the best way to take your mind off food.

It is now evening, and you have almost made it through your fasting day. This is the time to make sure you have had enough to drink throughout the day. The sun is not as bright right now, and it is a great time to go outside and do some gardening. Make overnight oats with 2 tablespoons of peanut butter, 1/2 cup of blueberries, and a small banana to eat in the morning.

Day 9

This morning to break your fast and eat the oats that you made the previous night. Remember to experiment with foods that you enjoy and mix them up a bit. If it is nice out, go outside and take a hike. Usually, you can find a park or something that offers some hiking. When doing any type of workout make sure you bring something healthy to drink. No sodas or other sugar-filled drinks; they tend to dehydrate you.

Have a farro salad for lunch today. Farro salads are excellent and healthy. They have a mix of farro, cucumber, roasted red bell peppers, chickpeas, olives, red onions, peppers, and Feta cheese. Farro is a mixture of multiple types of wheat. Like beans, these are sold dried, and they soften when cooked in water. With a mix of these vegetables and grains, you are likely to get most of your servings at lunch. Make sure to save some of the salad to use at a later date. Ensure you are getting enough fiber in your diet; it is vital for your health and helps you stay full throughout the day. After you have lunch, head out to the garden.

For the afternoon snack that tastes good, have 20 grams of kale chips. These are easy to make. You just need kale, olive oil, and salt, then bake it. Nothing could be simpler. Now stretch and relax with some yoga. If you start to lose a lot of hair, contact your doctor and stop fasting until you get the doctor's okay.

Tonight for dinner, thaw out some of that Italian white bean soup you froze a few days back for a fast and delicious dinner. Ensure you are diabetic to keep track of your sugar and check to make sure you are not going into ketosis. Go outside tonight and take a walk with a friend.

Day 10

Having a southwestern waffle is an excellent start to your day. Suppose you have never had one of these before you are in for a treat. It consists of a waffle, cooked egg, avocado, and sauce. When making food, it is important to measure out your ingredients to get an accurate calorie count. After breakfast, go outside and garden. Instead of having a handful of candy, opt for a piece of fruit. Some people call fruits nature's candies.

I am not a fan of any type of sushi that is not vegetarian. If you feel the same way, zucchini sushi is perfect for you. Nutritionists have recommended making lunch your largest meal of the day. After lunch, get together with a friend and do tai-chi. Activities done together are the most fun.

For a healthy but straightforward snack, have a medium-sized apple with 2 tablespoons of peanut butter. Once you are done with your snack, go out for a swim. I know not everyone has quick access to a pool. Many gyms now have it, and hotels too and just charge a small fee to let people who are not guests use it. Swimming is an exercise where you can quickly become dehydrated because you do not sweat or become hot while swimming.

Tonight, you can warm that split pea soup that you saved from earlier. Many exercises developed in the East are gentle, improve balance, and are excellent ways to relieve stress. If you are looking for more or fewer calories, you can add or take away from the food. An example would be at your snack time, add some almonds for a few more calories. For fewer calories, you could substitute the rice in the spiced pepper pilafs for cauliflower. After dinner, it is always nice to end your day with a nice walk.

Day 11 — fasting day

This morning change it a bit and go out for a short walk while enjoying your morning drink. When you are walking, you focus on things other than your hunger, which can help make your fasting time easier. By now, your body may have adjusted to fasting, where you no longer feel hungry on your fasting days.

Since earlier you went for a walk, it is time to do some weight lifting. If you have low blood pressure or low blood sugar, you need to make sure you feel well enough to work out. If you do not feel good when fasting, talk to your healthcare provider about other options.

Noon is the time you would typically have lunch; instead of eating, try to read a book, take a nap, or even a shower. If you have thought of combining Keto or some other eating plan with fasting, you may want to wait until your body is used to it.

During the afternoon, sit down and check out your journal. Do somebody's measurements so you can track your progress. Once you are done with your journaling, go outside and play some tennis with a friend. Make sure you are incorporating lentils in your diet a few times a week. Lentils are packed full of healthy nutrients.

In the evening, go out and take a walk with your dogs. Suppose you feel constipated, increase your water intake and find out if you are getting enough fiber in a day. After your walk, if you want to, you can go out in your garden. If you do not feel like it may be a hot shower will sound like a better way to end your night.

Day 12

Break your fast today with a parfait made with Ricotta cheese, yogurt, berries, chia seeds, and some almonds. Once you are eaten, try doing some pilates. This is similar to yoga with a few differences. Pilates focuses on resistant training and does an entire mat routine. If you have not had a change in your body or mental health, you may want to reevaluate what you are doing and see where you need to make changes.

Having a serving of cauliflower soup sounds like a good lunch. Cauliflower is another one of my favorite vegetables. I love having it steamed with some salt. Once you make your soup, sure to save some leftovers for dinner tomorrow night; once you are eaten, do 20 minutes of tai-chi. Make sure you are eating enough whole grains during the day.

A great afternoon snack is cherry tomatoes with Mozzarella cheese. Once you finish your snack, head out for some power walking for 30 minutes. Cardio workouts are essential for heart health.

For dinner, have a serving of apple salad with cinnamon and vinaigrette dressing. Once you eat, do yoga, then start meal planning for next week. Remember to keep in touch with family and friends. Do not focus entirely on going from one activity to the next. On your fasting days, you can go hang out with friends and do some shopping.

Day 13

Breakfast skillet hash is a great way to start your morning. Make sure you use Himalayan salt instead of table salt. Once you are ready, do some weight lifting. It sounds tedious, but weight lifting is a great way to gain muscle and tone your body.

Taco salad is such a great lunch. You can make it in many ways, and they all taste good. I have eaten taco salad for years, and I do not think any two have been the same. Fasting is one of the easiest ways to make a lifestyle change. After lunch, head out to the garden. There are times when you change the types of food you are eating. It can lead to depression and burnout. Be sure to watch out for that, and if you find yourself having these symptoms, it could be time to ease up a bit on your fasting schedule. This is one of the reasons it is essential to ease into fasting instead of jumping into it.

In the afternoon, you can have a small pear sliced with Ricotta cheese.

Once you finish your snack go out for a walk with a friend. This is just the start of your fasting journey and look at how far you have come. Now it is time to go through your food to see what you have to make meals for the next week and then write a list of the things you need.

Earlier this week, you had cauliflower soup today; pair up the soup with a serving of watercress salad. After dinner, spend some time meditating for at least 30 minutes. Focus on all areas of your body and check in how you are feeling.

Day 14

It is time to break your fast with a red berry smoothie. I love the smoothies; they are such a quick grab-and-go meal. After drinking your smoothie, try out another activity from the East called Qigong. It is very similar to tai-chi, and it is nice because almost anyone can do it. After working out, make sure you always have some protein.

Strawberry spinach salad is today's lunch. Make sure with all the extra workouts; you are getting your electrolytes. The best drink choices are coconut water or another type of natural sports drink. Being a natural type of drink is more important when you are not eating, so you do not break your fast. Today is a good time to go out in your garden or just look at how great it looks. When thinking about what to eat with intermittent fasting, think about easy and simple foods you already have at home.

A filling snack for the afternoon is cantaloupe slices wrapped in Prosciutto cheese. After your snack, see if one of your friends would like to play a game of badminton. If you want to keep track of your daily steps, feel motivated, and get a sense of accomplishment, get a pedometer.

Tonight's dinner will be broiled cheese stuffed portobellos. If you are not a fan of mushrooms, you can change the portobellos for a small-sized potato. After dinner, why not sit down and read a book or anything you find relaxing.

Now that you have finished your final week of the 2-step by step eating plans, how are you feeling? You can always alternate between the 2 programs anytime you feel like a change. With a total of 4 weeks under your belt, you should know most of the ins and outs of fasting. Your fasting time should have become much easier where you are not feeling hunger like you did during your first week.

If you are going to change your eating plan by adding a keto or Mediterranean diet to your fasting plan, you should be able to now.

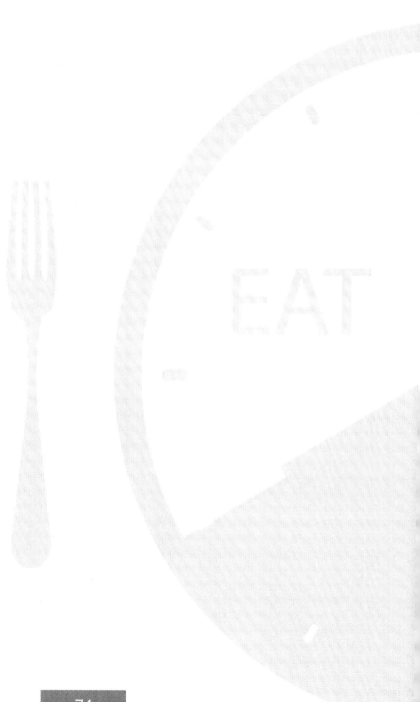

Conclusion

Thank you for getting to the end of the book, let's hope it was informative and able to provide you with all the tools you need to achieve your goals, whatever they may be.

Women over 50 have so many body changes going on and changes in hormones. It is hard to find a way to regain energy and become healthy, all while keeping our hormones level. The author, Nina Hodgson, had the same issues finding something to work when she turned 50. When she found fasting, she knew it was a whole new way of life and was excited to share it with others. She wrote her first book, "Intermittent Fasting for Women over 50: A Guide to Intermittent Fasting and Increasing Your Metabolism and Energy Levels. The Best Healthy Way to Detox Your Body and Rejuvenate" and knew she had to write another one because there is so much information to share, and she is excited to share it.

There is so much information out there about different ways to eat healthily. So many choices you can make and many diets to choose from. Fasting is the one that I have found to work the best. There are so many health benefits when using fasting as the start to a healthy

75

way of life. With fasting, you do not have to follow any type of eating plan. It is simply just eating and not eating for specific amounts of time and then making good choices — the benefits of fasting are endless. You can lose or gain weight depending on what you want to do. You will lower your blood pressure. Decrease your chances of diabetes, and reduce inflammation in your body.

Finally, if you found this book useful in any way, a review on Amazon is always appreciated!

Don't Forget my Gift!!!

Once again thanks for buying my book!. If you've read the book up to this point, I'm sure you appreciated the advice I wanted to share with you, so I'd be grateful if you'd like to share your appreciation too.

Leave a 5 star review:

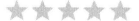

I ask you for an honest and truthful review.

This way you can help other women choose this book and embark on Intermittent Fasting.

Many thanks!

Click on the link below to get immediate access to

"The Intermittent Fasting Weekly Plan":

https://bit.ly/fastingweeklyplan

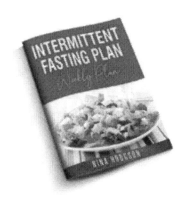